Infectious Diseases and Microbiology

nova
Medicine & Health
New York

Infectious Diseases and Microbiology

Psychological Consequences of the COVID-19 Pandemic on Children, Teenagers and Adults
Jean-Pascal Assailly, PhD
2022. ISBN: 978-1-68507-963-5 (Softcover)
2022. ISBN: 979-8-88697-072-2 (eBook)

Data Science Applications of Post-COVID-19 Psychological Disorders
Vijayalakshmi Kakulapati, PhD (Editor)
2022. ISBN: 979-8-88697-165-1 (Hardcover)
2022. ISBN: 979-8-88697-316-7 (eBook)

Interdisciplinary Approaches on Opportunistic Infections and Future Prospects
Jayapradha Ramakrishnan, PhD
and Ganesh Babu Malli Mohan, PhD (Editors)
2022. ISBN: 978-1-68507-984-0 (Softcover)
2022. ISBN: 979-8-88697-342-6 (eBook)

A Closer Look at the COVID-19 Variants
Richard D. Hylton (Editor)
2022. ISBN: 979-8-88697-170-5 (Hardcover)
2022. ISBN: 979-8-88697-221-4 (eBook)

COVID-19: Vaccines, Testing and Compensation Programs
Mark N. Frierson (Editor)
2022. ISBN: 979-8-88697-167-5 (Hardcover)
2022. ISBN: 979-8-88697-220-7 (eBook)

More information about this series can be found at
https://novapublishers.com/product-category/series/infectious-diseases-and-microbiology/

Yvette S. Brewer
Editor

Infectious Diseases

From Prevention to Control

nova
Medicine & Health
New York

Library of Congress Cataloging-in-Publication Data

ISBN: 979-8-88697-657-1

Published by Nova Science Publishers, Inc. † New York

Contents

Preface	... vii
Chapter 1	**Solid Lipid Nanoparticles as Innovative Strategies for the Treatment and Prophylaxis of Infectious Diseases** ... 1 C. Rodríguez Laboccetta, A. Videla Garrido, V. Briceño Fernández, M. A. Toscanini, A. D. Nusblat and M. L. Cuestas
Chapter 2	**An Agent-Based Model of Infectious Diseases That Incorporates the Roles of Immune Cells and Antibodies** ... 123 Shigeaki Ogibayashi
Chapter 3	**Endophytic Actinobacteria: A Source of Novel Bioactive Metabolites for the Treatment of Infectious Diseases** ... 171 Juri Saikia, Rajkumari Mazumdar and Debajit Thakur
Chapter 4	**Infectious Diseases: Antibiotic Resistance and Stewardship** ... 197 Rajkumari Mazumdar, Juri Saikia and Debajit Thakur
Index	... 219

Preface

This book contains four selected chapters on infectious diseases, covering topics from prevention to control. Chapter One examines the potential of solid lipid nanoparticles to act as innovative treatment and prophylaxis options for infectious diseases. Chapter Two provides an agent-based model of infectious diseases that incorporates the roles of immune cells and antibodies. Chapter Three is an overview of endophytic actinobacteria as a source of novel bioactive metabolites for the treatment of infectious diseases. Chapter Four examines the issue of antibiotic resistance and stewardship that faces humanity at this time.

Chapter 1 - Despite the advances in the understanding of the pathogenesis of infectious diseases and the development of novel treatments and vaccines to control and prevent them, these pathogenic disorders are among the most common causes of hospitalization and death worldwide.

Nanotechnology has recently emerged as a promising tool in biomedicine research. An important branch of nanotechnology is drug delivery and drug targeting using a wide range of biomaterials with auspicious potential applications in numerous infectious diseases.

Solid lipid nanoparticles (SLNs) have emerged as carriers for therapeutic drugs, peptides, proteins, antigens and bioactive molecules, as well as for vaccine delivery. They are made up of a solid matrix that allows the controlled release of the drug or other molecules accommodated between fatty acid chains. A review of the nanomaterials used for the preparation of SLNs will be summarized. The current state-of-the art on several SLN formulations as nanocarriers of FDA-approved drugs for the therapy and prophylaxis of various infectious diseases, including those considered neglected by the World Health Organization that are under preclinical or clinical trials, will be addressed in this chapter.

Chapter 2 - In this study, an agent-based infection model focusing on recovery process modeling was constructed and the following results were obtained. The present model well reproduced the qualitative features of the chronological pattern in the numbers of newly infected, newly recovered, and total infected agents observed in the real world. The factors of the model that are indispensable for reproducing the actual pandemic are the roles of fever and antibodies, which increase the upper limit of the rate of virus replication for pandemic convergence. The role of fever is modeled as the effect of immunity increasing with an increasing number of viruses, and the role of antibodies is modeled as antibodies emerging when the immunity is insufficient to keep up with virus replication.

The critical factor determining whether pandemic convergence occurs is whether the system includes severely infected agents whose immune response cannot keep up with the virus replication rate. Such severely infected agents are characterized by a high body temperature and a massive number of viruses. To control infection spread, it is essential to identify infected individuals, especially severely infected ones, and isolate them from the system. Measuring body temperature is effective in identifying severely infected individuals, rather than PCR tests, because fever is a sign of being infected and also provides information about the severity of infection, while PCR tests provide information only in a dichotomous positive/negative format.

To overcome the pandemic while minimizing the economic impact, it is effective to identify and isolate infected individuals by monitoring body temperature and refusing entry of those infected at national borders, such as airports, and also in densely populated places. It is also effective for individuals to determine their own infection status by monitoring their own body temperature. Wearing masks and providing ventilation in densely populated spaces are also effective because they decrease the number of viruses at the time of infection.

Chapter 3 - The emergence of infectious diseases has put on an alarming threat to human health and progress. The World Health Organization (WHO) claims that infectious diseases continue to spread and emerge and that efforts being made globally to combat newly emerging and drug-resistant infections are jeopardized by a lack of new antimicrobials (2020). COVID-19, a recent pandemic that has affected the entire world and claimed the lives of 2.7 million people, has hundreds of millions of documented cases (2021). Outbreaks of infectious disease can have detrimental social, political, and economic ramifications, and emerging and overlooking infectious diseases pose a real threat to public health.

Since the historic IOM report that emphasized the significance of emerging infectious diseases, much has been taught from previous outbreaks and significant strides have been made. Yet, preparing for pandemics continues to be a significant global challenge. It has been discovered that a wide range of factors, including human behavior and activities, pathogen evolution, poverty, environmental changes, and dynamic human interactions with animals, all contributed to the emergence and spread of infectious diseases. Furthermore, the emergence of pathogens that are resistant to antibiotics has reduced the number of available treatments and caused incurable infections, necessitating the development of novel antibiotics.

There is a global need to find novel sources of antibiotics. Natural products produced by endophytic actinobacteria (EA) act as a source of potential new antibiotics. In addition, they seem to be a source of brand-new, potent compounds to fight the rising tide of pathogens with multidrug resistance. Endophytic actinobacteria reside within plant tissues and interact with the host to produce diverse bioactive metabolites. Exploration of endophytic actinobacteria from untouched ecosystems is going on in the search for new bioactive molecules. The current review highlights the isolation and discovery of potent novel bioactive metabolites produced by endophytic actinobacteria associated with diverse ecosystems.

Chapter 4 - Infectious diseases are illnesses caused by pathogenic microorganisms that enter our bodies from the outside. They can sometimes be caught by other people, the environment, animal contact, or insect bites. Some infections are so mild that we might not notice any symptoms, while others can be fatal. Existing and emerging infectious diseases pose significant challenges to public health outcomes around the globe. Pathogenic bacteria continue to be a severe health concern, causing many fatalities and hospitalizations yearly. Due to the development of new variants of drug-resistant pathogenic microorganisms, the treatment and immunization of infectious diseases have become even more challenging in recent years. Existing diagnostic techniques are inefficient because they lack speed and ultra-sensitivity. Therefore, novel therapeutic and diagnostic approaches are required.

The primary goal of this study is to highlight current trends in antibiotic resistance as well as novel therapeutic prospects for future disease management and control advancements.

Chapter 1

Solid Lipid Nanoparticles as Innovative Strategies for the Treatment and Prophylaxis of Infectious Diseases

C. Rodríguez Laboccetta[1,2], A. Videla Garrido[2], V. Briceño Fernández[1,2], M. A. Toscanini[1,2], A. D. Nusblat[1] and M. L. Cuestas[2,*]

[1] University of Buenos Aires, CONICET,
Institute of Nanobiotechnology (NANOBIOTEC),
Buenos Aires, Argentina
[2] University of Buenos Aires, CONICET,
Research Institute in Microbiology and Medical Parasitology (IMPaM),
Buenos Aires, Argentina

Abstract

Despite the advances in the understanding of the pathogenesis of infectious diseases and the development of novel treatments and vaccines to control and prevent them, these pathogenic disorders are among the most common causes of hospitalization and death worldwide.

Nanotechnology has recently emerged as a promising tool in biomedicine research. An important branch of nanotechnology is drug delivery and drug targeting using a wide range of biomaterials with auspicious potential applications in numerous infectious diseases.

Solid lipid nanoparticles (SLNs) have emerged as carriers for therapeutic drugs, peptides, proteins, antigens and bioactive molecules, as well as for vaccine delivery. They are made up of a solid matrix that allows the controlled release of the drug or other molecules

---

* Corresponding Author's Email: marilucuestas@gmail.com.

In: Infectious Diseases
Editor: Yvette S. Brewer
ISBN: 979-8-88697-657-1

accommodated between fatty acid chains. A review of the nanomaterials used for the preparation of SLNs will be summarized. The current state-of-the art on several SLN formulations as nanocarriers of FDA-approved drugs for the therapy and prophylaxis of various infectious diseases, including those considered neglected by the World Health Organization that are under preclinical or clinical trials, will be addressed in this chapter.

Keywords: infectious diseases, neglected tropical diseases, solid lipid nanoparticles, sustained drug release, targeted drug delivery, biomaterials, vaccines

Introduction

Despite all the advances in elucidating the mechanisms by which pathogens cause disease as well as in the development of many therapeutic tools to combat infection, infectious diseases are among the top 10 causes of death worldwide [1]. According to the World Health Organization (WHO), of the 55.4 million deaths around the world in 2019, lower respiratory infections were the most deadly communicable diseases, with 2.6 million deaths, followed by diarrheal diseases (1.5 million deaths) and tuberculosis (TB) (1.5 million deaths). In low-income countries, the number of deaths caused by infectious diseases is significantly higher than in high-income countries. For instance, in low-income countries it was reported that almost 80 deaths per 100,000 inhabitants were due to low respiratory infections, whereas in high-income countries this rate was lower (less than 60 deaths per 100,000 inhabitants) [1]. This means that developing countries face a great challenge in combating infection diseases since many people still do not have access to antimicrobials, and any failure to control their spread, would also represent a hazard to developed countries. In addition, the emergence of multi-drug resistant pathogens makes this scenario even bleaker since it limits the utility of current therapies against infection diseases, leading to an increased morbidity and mortality, longer hospital stays, and severe economic loss to patients and nations [2].

Thus, resistance to the drugs used to treat numerous bacterial, viral, fungal and protozoan infections, such as TB, HIV/AIDS, invasive candidiasis and malaria is a serious matter of health concern. Recently, extensive drug-resistance (XDR) and pandrug-resistance (PDR) among Gram-negative bacterial and mycobacterial infections have been documented worldwide [3];

however, in this chapter all these terms will be used indistinctly as multi-drug resistance (MDR) to avoid confusion. In 2019, the Interagency Coordination Group on Antimicrobial Resistance reported that MDR diseases had already caused at least 700,000 global annual deaths, including 230,000 deaths from MDR TB, a figure that could increase to 10 million deaths globally per year by 2050 if no action is taken. The economic damage of uncontrolled MDR could be as high as that experienced during the 2008-2009 global financial crisis owing to increased health care costs, impact on food and feed production, trade and livelihoods, and increased poverty and inequality [4].

At present, the emergence of MDR represents a frightening hazard to patients infected with this kind of pathogens since no "magic bullet" is available to overcome this issue, making MDR a similar condition that existed during the pre-antibiotic era as common diseases are now becoming untreatable [5].

This stark reality is considered a global crisis that threatens a century of progress in controlling disease and health. Lifesaving medical procedures such as surgeries, transplantations, care of critically ill or immunocompromised patients are becoming riskier to be performed due to the absence of effective antimicrobial agents to combat MDR pathogens. The slogan adopted by the WHO in 2011 "No action today, no cure tomorrow" clearly shows the need to act immediately and start combating MDR [6].

Another major issue is related to the role of microbial biofilms in several human infections. Biofilms are considered an alternative lifestyle in which microorganisms adopt a multicellular behavior that facilitates and/or prolongs survival in diverse environmental niches [7]. In vents and biomedical devices, the formation of biofilms enables pathogens to persist for long periods of time as reservoirs that can potentially spread to patients [8]. Inside the host, biofilms allow pathogens to evade innate immune responses, and are thus associated with long-term persistence and chronic infections such as pneumonia in cystic fibrosis patients, non-healing chronic wounds, chronic otitis media, periodontitis, osteomyelitis, kidney infections, endocarditis and implant- and catheter-associated infections [9]. According to the National Institute of Health, biofilms account for up to 80% of the total number of microbial infections [10]. Biofilms are particularly refractory to antimicrobial treatments, due to diffusion limitations exerted by the extracellular matrix, antimicrobial inactivation by high metal ion concentration and low pH, and the presence of metabolically inactive persistent cells that survive treatment, but also because of an increased transmission of resistance markers within the biofilm community as was widely described in bacteria [11]. Combined, these attributes make, for instance, biofilm bacteria up to 1,000-fold more tolerant and/or resistant to antibiotics than planktonic cells [12].

Another important point is related to the ability of the infectious agent to produce intracellular infections (e.g., viruses, *Mycoplasma* spp., *Mycobacterium* spp., *Histoplasma capsulatum*, *Chlamydia* spp., *Brucella abortus*, *Listeria monocytogenes*, *Salmonella enterica*, *Trypanosoma cruzi*, *Toxoplasma gondii, Leishmania* spp.). These intracellular infections are difficult to eradicate due to low availability and activity of anti-infective drugs inside cells, turning them into reservoirs. Furthermore, some drugs display limited bioavailability in the target microorganism to exert their therapeutic effect.

Finally, a large number of antimicrobial drugs (almost 50%) display low solubility in biological fluids, being this issue still the main limitation in oral, parenteral, and transdermal administration [13].

Thus, there is an urgent need for better treatment strategies that can (i) improve the activity of the existing antimicrobial drugs by anatomic targeting or by enhancing bioavailability, stability and aqueous solubility of drugs, (ii) enhance the antimicrobial activity against biofilms and (iii) actively overcome the MDR phenotype in both pathogens and host cells, depending on the pathogenesis of the infectious agent.

Nanotechnology is a young field that has evolved as a technology with direct applications in medicine, offering the potential for designing and developing novel devices and therapeutic platforms within a nanometer range capable of improving clinical outcomes [14]. Doxil™, AmBisome™, Abraxane™, Arikayce™ and Onpattro™ are just five examples of the potential of nanotechnology to achieve therapeutic success. In addition, the Pfizer-BioNTech COVID-19 Vaccine (COMIRNATY™) and the Moderna COVID-19 vaccine (Spikevax™), the two mRNA-COVID 19 vaccines approved by the Food and Drug Administration (FDA) in 2021, are based on lipid nanoparticles, which have held a recognized position in the mainstream of drug delivery systems since the discovery of liposomes in the 1960s.

Photodynamic therapy, gene therapy, immunotherapy, vaccinology, cancer therapy, antimicrobial therapy, imaging techniques and diagnosis are the clinical areas that were most revolutionized by nanotechnology [13]. Recently, its application to infectious diseases was reflected by the emergence of innovative approaches that enable their prevention, diagnosis and treatment (e.g., sustained drug release to avoid lifetime antimicrobial therapies, drug delivery via oral, parenteral, transdermal and pulmonary routes, vaccine delivery, drug targeting at specific cellular and organ levels and microbicides) [15-24].

As mentioned above, nanotechnology has the power to radically change the chemo-resistance nature induced to host cells by some pathogens (e.g., HIV [25]) by overcoming the MDR phenotype related to the overexpression of several members of the ATP-binding cassette (ABC)-transporters superfamily, such as P-gp or MDR1 that efflux drugs out of cells decreasing their efficacy [26, 27]. Other approaches using nanotechnology to combat MDR include [28]:

I. Nanoparticles with multiple antimicrobial mechanisms, e.g., reactive oxygen species (ROS)-generator nanoparticles, more specifically RNOS (reactive nitrogen oxide species) and metal-based nanoparticles, including formulations with silver (Ag), zinc (Zn), copper (Cu), titanium (Ti), magnesium (Mg), and gold (Au).
II. Multiple antimicrobial drugs with different therapeutic targets or mechanisms of action in one nanoparticle.
III. Nanoparticles that can reduce biofilm formation, and combat intracellular microorganisms.
IV. Nanoparticles that encapsulate antimicrobial agents for targeted drug delivery to administer higher doses at the infected site, thereby overcoming resistance with fewer adverse effects in patients.

SLNs could impact the latter three points to improve the efficacy of antimicrobial agents because they can (i) encapsulate multiple drugs; (ii) increase the intracellular uptake of drugs, and (iii) be modified for active or passive targeting upon reaching the affected site to deliver the drug [29-31].

SLNs are also useful in reducing toxicity and improving the oral bioavailability of drugs, as will be described in Section 4.

The present chapter will especially focus on infectious diseases, with particular emphasis on neglected tropical diseases (NTDs) and nanotechnology, highlighting current efforts to develop new ways of treating infections and improving pharmacotherapy. In particular, the application of solid lipid nanoparticle (SLN) formulations for the delivery of commercially available drugs, and future challenges using these innovative tools are addressed, including preclinical and clinical studies. A description of the biomaterials used to prepare SLNs is also thoroughly discussed.

This chapter is organized into 5 sections. Section 1 is an introductory section. Section 2 addresses infectious diseases and NTDs. Section 3 is concerned with nanotechnology and nanomedicines. Section 4 sheds light on different aspects of SLNs, including their advantages and disadvantages for drug encapsulation and release, methods of preparation and characterization, biomaterials and formulation variables. This section also analyzes the role of SLNs in the delivery of antifungal, antiviral, antiparasitic and antibacterial drugs, as well as the current status of SLNs in vaccine formulations, addressing the preclinical and clinical studies. Section 5 concludes this chapter with general remarks.

The Unseen World: From Magical and Divine Explanations of Disease to Infectious Diseases and NTDs

Whether attributed to the anger of the gods, unbalanced energies, demons, witchcrafts or exposure to poisonous vapors or miasmas, infectious diseases have been an undesired companion that evoked fear and awe among human civilizations since time immemorial, decimating populations through pandemics and everyday difficult-to-treat infections [32]. "The Antonine Plague" (or "The Plague of Galen," 165-180 A.D.), "The plague of Justinian" (541-542 A.D.), "The Black Death" (or "The plague," 1347-1351 A.D.), "The Spanish Flu" (or "The Spanish Lady," 1918-1919 A.D.), and HIV/AIDS (1981-present) are among the five worst devastating pandemics that had deeply affected humanity. Nowadays, the coronavirus disease 2019 (COVID-19) pandemic caused by the severe acute respiratory syndrome coronavirus 2 (SARS-CoV-2) has pushed the world into a substantial health, social, economic and political crisis with 615,310,890 confirmed cases, 6,524,568 deaths and 12,677,499,928 vaccine doses administered at the time this chapter was being prepared [33]. This world-breaking record in vaccine development and mass immunization show the crucial potential that mRNA vaccines have in responding to new epidemics and even pandemics.

Great advances have been achieved since the first discovery of protists and bacteria by Antoine van Leeuwenhoek, who described these unicellular organisms as 'animalcules' in his famous "letter on the protozoa" in 1677 [34] and the subsequent demonstration by the Nobel Laureate in Medicine and founder of the science of bacteriology, Robert Koch, with his famous Koch´s postulates formulated along with Friederich Loeffler, establishing that certain microorganisms are the cause of major human diseases. It was in the second half of the 19th century that microbiology began its golden age, sweeping away doubts about the existence and importance of microorganisms. During a period of 20 years, the main bacterial agents that caused disease in humans and animals were discovered, improvements in hygiene were achieved and the field of immunology evolved, leading to the development of serological tests for diagnosis, vaccines for preventing infectious diseases and drugs for therapy [35].

Edward Jenner, and the smallpox vaccination, Ignaz Semmelweiss and his antiseptic procedures; Louis Pasteur and his major breakthroughs in the causes and prevention of diseases; Joseph Lister and the introduction of sterile surgery by using aseptic methods; Paul Ehrlich and his magic bullets in chemotherapy, and Alexander Fleming and his discovery of penicillin that paved the way for the development of modern antibiotics, are among the greatest scientists of all times that revolutionized the history of microbiology. As a result of these major milestones in microbiology research, the human burden of infectious diseases has been significantly reduced, and at present, small-pox is fully eradicated with polio set to hopefully follow thanks to the large-scale administration of their respective smallpox and oral polio vaccines [36]. In this connection, wild poliovirus types 2 and 3 have been successfully eradicated and wild poliovirus type 1 is endemic in only two countries - Pakistan and Afghanistan.

Some nefarious events that overshadow all the progress achieved so far includes the emergence of new diseases (for example, SARS, MERS, COVID-19, monkeypox, Langya henipavirus), the evolution of MDR pathogens, the re-emergence of infectious diseases that have been under control by mass immunization programs (i.e., measles, circulating vaccine-derived poliovirus (cVDPV) type 2 – which accounts for more than 90% of current cVDPV outbreaks, and which poses a major challenge to achieving global polio eradication), the widespread in some geographical regions of known pathogens that have persisted in natural reservoirs mostly unnoticed, such as the *Hantaan virus* in South America, the filovirus *Ebola virus* (EBOV) and *Marburg virus* (MBV) in Africa or the arboviruses *Zika virus* (ZV), *Dengue virus* (DENV), *Chikungunya virus* (CHIKV) and *Yellow fever virus* (YFV) in tropical and subtropical regions of the world [36].

At present, more than 1,400 species of infectious agents have been shown to cause disease in humans, including pathogens for some 347 diseases of sustained clinical importance. Of them, 110 pose a threat to non-immune travelers and 62 can be prevented by vaccination -19 usually as routine childhood immunizations [37]. Twenty diseases are considered NTDs by the WHO, being them a group of communicable diseases that are prevalent in tropical and subtropical areas of 149 countries [38]. It is estimated that more than 1 billion people are currently affected, particularly, populations living in poverty, often stigmatized and excluded from society, without access to safe water, adequate sanitation and basic health services that may also live in close contact with infectious vectors and domestic animals or livestock [39]. The main features of these diseases are shown in Table 1. Local epidemiological studies and the availability of appropriate measures to detect, prevent and control such diseases is a way to control and potentially eradicate them.

In this regard, combatting infectious diseases, and in particular NDTs and MDR, remains a high priority in the twenty-first century and requires intra and interdisciplinary approaches and planned investments aiming to track, prevent, diagnose, treat infection and ultimately reduce poverty and improve the health and social well-being of affected populations.

The field of infectious disease therapeutics is evolving very quickly. It is highly necessary to use medical, scientific, pharmaceutical and technological knowledge to address the socioeconomic and health burden resulting from conditions such as NDTs and MDR. Regretfully, the extremely high cost of novel pharmacotherapies for combatting infectious diseases preclude their implementation mainly in developing countries and less affluent populations.

In the last few years, nanotechnology has contributed to improving the administration and delivery of many drugs. A number of reasons support the fact that nanotechnologies can provide unique solutions also in poorer societies, including those from Africa, Asia and South America [40]:

- Strong nanotechnology research in developing countries oriented to the solution of specific therapeutic problems of their own communities will make these new technologies more affordable.
- Increasing funding by public and private organizations for research on specific diseases affecting primarily the developing world.
- Anatomical and cellular targeting using nanotechnology could improve therapeutic success by reducing adverse effects through decreasing the frequency of administration regimens, increasing patient compliance, and reducing treatment costs substantially. In addition, drug-targeting can increase its effectiveness and even extend its applicability by overcoming some technological limitations (e.g., low bioavailability), resistance, anatomical and cellular barriers, among others.

Table 1. Neglected tropical diseases and their main features

Disease	Causative agent	Main characteristics	Prevalence	Therapy	Prophylaxis
Buruli ulcer	*Mycobacterium ulcerans*	Bacterial necrotizing cutaneous disease distributed mainly in West and Central Africa and other tropical countries. The exotoxin mycolactone of *M. ulcerans* is the main virulence factor of the infection that causes skin lesions, nodules or ulcers. Early diagnosis and treatment are critical to reduce morbidity and prevent long-term disability.	2,217 cases were reported worldwide in 2017.	Rifampicin and streptomycin.	Avoid risky activities (swimming, fishing, agricultural works, etc.) in endemic areas.
Chagas disease	*Trypanosoma cruzi*	Parasitic anthropozoonosis endemic in Latin America and spread worldwide. Transmitted mainly by vector (*Triatoma, Panstrongylus, Rhodnius*) and to a lesser extent congenitally and horizontally through blood transfusion and organ transplantation. Around 30–40% of chronic infected people suffer from cardiomyopathy, arrhythmias, hepatosplenomegaly, and, less frequently, polyneuropathy and stroke.	Around 5.7 million infected people in Latin America in 2010.	Benznidazole as first-line treatment or nifurtimox.	Vector control programs and blood screening.

Table 1. (Continued)

Disease	Causative agent	Main characteristics	Prevalence	Therapy	Prophylaxis
Dengue and Chikungunya	Dengue virus serotypes 1–4 (DENV) Chikungunya virus (CHIKV)	Arthropod-borne viral diseases endemic in every global region except for continental Europe. Transmitted mainly by mosquitos of the species *Aedes aegypti* and *Aedes albopictus.* Infection by DENV is mostly asymptomatic, but a spectrum of disease ranging from self-limited fever to life-threatening shock can be produced. In contrast, most people infected with CHIKV present febrile illness characterized by severe arthralgias.	Dengue: 390 million infected people in 2013. Chikungunya: Around 123,000 confirmed cases in America in 2017.	Supportive treatment. Acetaminophen is preferred for pain and fever control over non-steroidal anti-inflammatory drugs.	Dengvaxia® (recombinant vaccine - chimeric yellow fever virus-DENV tetravalent dengue vaccine). Personal protection measures to avoid mosquito bites.
Dracunculiasis (guinea-worm disease)	*Dracunculus medinensis*	Parasitic disease endemic to rural and low-income areas of the world, mostly African countries. Transmitted by drinking water contaminated with crustacean copepods infected with the larvae of the parasite. When the adult worm emerges through the skin approximately one year after infection, it can cause blistering, ulceration, edema and pruritus. Cellulitis, sepsis or abscess can also occur.	25 infected people until June 2019.	Supportive treatment. Anti-inflammatory agents for pain and topical antibiotic cream or systemic antibiotics for bacterial infection.	Drink safe water or filtered drinking water in endemic regions.

Disease	Causative agent	Main characteristics	Prevalence	Therapy	Prophylaxis
Echinococcosis	*Echinococcus granulosus* (cystic echinococcosis), *E. multilocularis* (alveolar echinococcosis), *E. vogeli* (polycystic echinococcosis) and *E. oligarthrus* (unicystic echinococcosis)	Parasitic disease with four distinguished forms: cystic (CE), alveolar (AE), polycystic (PE) and unicystic (UE). CE is globally distributed and highly endemic in rural areas of South America, Central Asia, North and East Africa and the Mediterranean. AE is confined to the Northern Hemisphere. CE and AE are the most common forms and can cause serious morbidity and death. Humans become infected by ingestion of food and water contaminated with the parasite eggs or by close contact with an infected animal, generally dogs and livestock.	>1 million people are affected globally each year.	CE: Depending on a variety of factors the treatment could be administration of benzimidazole or mebendazole, surgery or percutaneous treatment with the PAIR technique (Puncture, aspiration, injection and reaspiration) AE: surgery followed by albendazole.	Health education, periodic dog deworming and sheep vaccination.
Foodborne trematodiases	• Clonorchis sinensis (Clonorchiasis) • *Fasciola hepatica* and *F. gigantica* (fascioliasis) • *Opisthorchis viverrini and O. felineus* (opisthorchiasis) • Paragonimus spp (Paragonimiasis)	Clonorchiasis and opisthorchiasis: fish-borne liver flukes endemic in Asia and Estern Europe. Humans become infected by ingestion of raw, undercooked or poorly processed fish contaminated with metacercariae. Infections may be asymptomatic or mildly symptomatic but patients with a very high worm burden may have fever and right upper-quadrant pain.	Estimated infected people worldwide: • Clonorchis sinensis: 601 million • Fasciolasis: 2.4-17 million • Opisthorchiasis: 11.2 million • Paragonimiasis: 20.7 million	• Clonorchis sinensis, Opisthorchiasis, Paragonimiasis: Praziquantel • Fasciolasis: triclabendazol	Safe food practices and veterinary public health measures.

Table 1. (Continued)

Disease	Causative agent	Main characteristics	Prevalence	Therapy	Prophylaxis
		Severe and chronic infection may cause obstructive jaundice, cirrhosis, cholangitis, acalculous cholecystitis, bile peritonitis or cholangiocarcinoma. Fasciolasis: Parasitic disease of worldwide distribution. Humans become infected by ingestion of contaminated plants, mainly watercress, or water. Once the parasite infects the liver, there is an incubation period followed by an acute or invasive phase, then a latency period of months or years, and finally a chronic or obstructive phase. Paragonimiasis: lung fluke disease endemic in Central and South America, Asia and Africa. Humans become infected by ingestion of raw or undercooked freshwater crabs, crayfish and other crustaceans. Symptoms include hemorrhage, chronic cough, dyspnea, fever, and necrosis of the lung parenchyma. Complications such as pleural effusion and pneumothorax can occur.			

Disease	Causative agent	Main characteristics	Prevalence	Therapy	Prophylaxis
Human African trypanosomiasis (sleeping sickness)	*Trypanosoma brucei gambiense* and *Trypanosoma brucei rhodesiense*	Parasitic disease endemic in intertropical Africa transmitted by the bite of tsetse flies (Diptera, genus *Glossina*). While *T. brucei gambiense* is the most prevalent subspecies, *T. brucei rhodesiense* only affects humans sporadically. The disease progresses from a hemolymphatic stage to a second–stage characterized by central nervous system invasion with neurological disorders, such as sleep disturbances.	2,164 reported cases in 2016.	*T brucei gambiense* 1st stage: pentamidine isethionate. 2nd stage: eflornithine combined with nifurtimox PO *T. brucei rhodesiense* 1st stage: suramin 2nd stage: melarsoprol	Vector control and control of the animal reservoir.
Leishmaniasis	*Leishmania* spp.	Parasitic group of vector-borne diseases that mainly affect poor people of the Mediterranean Basin, East Africa, America and Southeast Asia. Humans become infected by the bites of infected sandflies (*Phlebotomus or Lutzomyia*). Most people infected remain asymptomatic; however, when infection progresses various clinical manifestations with different degrees of severity are observed depending on parasite characteristics, vector biology, and host factors.	22,145 reported cases in 2017.	Pentavalent antimony as first-line drug. Pentamidine and amphotericin as second-line drugs.	Vector control (indoor residual spraying, long-lasting insecticidal nets, and environmental management).

Table 1. (Continued)

Disease	Causative agent	Main characteristics	Prevalence	Therapy	Prophylaxis
		There are three main forms of the disease: cutaneous, mucocutaneous and life-threatening visceral form.			
Leprosy (Hansen's disease)	*Mycobacterium leprae*	Chronic bacterial disease endemic in Southeast Asia, America, Africa, Western Pacific, and Eastern Mediterranean. The disease mainly affects the skin, peripheral nerves, mucosal surfaces of the upper respiratory tract and eyes. Transmission occurs by respiratory droplets but the exact transmission mechanism has not yet been entirely elucidated. While around 90%-95% of infected people are asymptomatic, the disease presentation in the remaining 10% depends on patient's genetic factors. Skin infection produces cutaneous manifestations and neurologic infection causes sensory loss, disability and deformity. Eyes, mucous membranes, testes and bones can also be affected.	210,973 infected people worldwide in 2017.	Multidrug therapy with rifampicin, clofazimine and dapsone.	Single dose rifampicin as post-exposure prophylaxis after contact with leprosy patients.

Disease	Causative agent	Main characteristics	Prevalence	Therapy	Prophylaxis
Lymphatic filariasis	*Wuchereria bancrofti, Brugia malayi* and *B. timori*	Parasitic mosquito-borne disease endemic throughout the tropics and subtropics of Africa, Asia, the western Pacific and some regions of the Caribbean and South America. Parasite larvae are transmitted by the bite of mosquitos of the gender *Aedes, Anopheles, Culex, Mansonia, and Ochlerotatus*. Generally, infected individuals remain asymptomatic but with underlying lymphatic damage. The infection then leads to acute attacks, lymphedema and elephantiasis or hydrocele. The disease causes permanent disfigurement and chronic disability.	120 million infected people worldwide.	• Albendazole with ivermectin • Albendazole plus diethyl-carbamazine • Diethylcarbamazine citrate (DEC)	• Personal protection measures to avoid mosquito bites. • Vector control • Mass drug administration of h albendazole plus ivermectin or DEC. to the risk population
Mycetoma, chromoblastomycosis and other deep mycoses	Actinomycetoma(*): • *Norcardia brasiliensis* • *Actinomadure Madura* • *Streptomyces somaliensis* • *Actinomadura pelletieri* Eumycetoma(*): • *Madurella mycetomatis*	Mycetoma: mutilating, chronic and granulomatous infection of the subcutaneous tissue caused by the traumatic inoculation of aerobic actinomycetic bacteria (actinomycetoma) or fungi (eumycetoma). Nowadays, at least 56 different microorganisms are believed to be responsible agents for mycetoma. This disease is characterized by numerous deformations, disabilities and could be potentially fatal.	As they are not notifiable diseases, information regarding prevalence is lacking. In Sudán, a prevalence of 14.5 per 1000 population was reported in 2010.	Actinomycetoma: • Co-trimoxazole and amikacin • Eumycetoma: • Itraconazole and cryosurgery Chromoblastomycosis: • Cryosurgery • Itraconazole • Voriconazole • Posaconazole	Avoid traumatic fungal or bacteria inoculation, Disinfect wounds and wear shoes.

Table 1. (Continued)

Disease	Causative agent	Main characteristics	Prevalence	Therapy	Prophylaxis
	Chromoblastomycosis (*): • *Fonsecaea pedrosoi* • *Cladophialophora carrionii* *Phialophora verrucosa*	The "mycetoma belt" is the region between latitudes 15° S and 30° N in which most cases occur. Chromoblastomycosis: chronic fungal infection of cutaneous and subcutaneous tissues with nodular, verrucous and tumoral lesions. Tropical and subtropical climates are the most common in which the infection occurs, specifically in rural areas. Pigmented or dematiaceous saprophytic moulds ubiquitous in the environment are the main causative agents. A non-protective T helper type 2 (Th2) immune response with ineffective humoral involvement and the presence of muriform cells encrusted in the infected tissue are characteristic signs. Endemic in tropical and subtropical regions of the planet, between latitudes 30° N and 30°S.		• Combination of itraconazole plus terbinafine	

Disease	Causative agent	Main characteristics	Prevalence	Therapy	Prophylaxis
Onchocerciasis (river blindness)	*Onchocerca volvulus*	Infectious disease transmitted from person to person by the repeated bites of infected black flies (*Simulium* spp.) with the filarial worms of *O. volvulus*. Symptoms are subcutaneous nodules, severe itching, pruritus, skin atrophy, skin pigmentation and blindness.After trachoma, it is the second cause of blindness due to infection	37 million people infected worldwide.	Ivermectin	Mass-treatment programs using ivermectin.
Rabies	*Lyssaviruses*	Viral zoonotic disease that is usually transmitted to humans by animal bites. It causes progressive and fatal inflammation of the brain and spinal cord. There are encephalitic and paralytic forms of the disease. The infection is always fatal after clinical disease develops. Approximately 99% rabies cases are acquired from the bite of an infected dog.	Causes 59,000 human deaths annually in over 150 countries.	Not available	Wound cleansing, administration of rabies vaccine and rabies immune globulin.
Scabies and other ectoparasites	*Sarcoptes scabiei var hominis*	Contagious skin infestation transmitted primarily through person-to-person contact. Symptoms are debilitating itching, reduced ability to concentrate, social stigmatization and ongoing health care expenses. This infestation may be complicated by bacterial infection which may cause septicemia, heart disease and chronic kidney disease.	130 million people affected worldwide.	• Permethrin • Ivermectin • Antihistamines to control itchiness	Mass-treatment programs using topical permethrin or oral ivermectin.

Table 1. (Continued)

Disease	Causative agent	Main characteristics	Prevalence	Therapy	Prophylaxis
Schistosomiasis	Schistosomes	Infectious disease of poverty that leads to chronic ill-health. It is prevalent in tropical and subtropical areas, in communities lacking potable water and suitable sanitation. Infection is acquired by ingestion of water infested with the larval forms of parasitic blood flukes. There are two major forms: urogenital schistosomiasis that causes hematuria and may lead to infertility, and intestinal schistosomiasis produces abdominal pain, diarrhea and blood in the stool. Symptoms in children include anemia, stunted growth and reduced ability to learn.	240 million people affected worldwide.	• Praziquantel (safe in pregnancy and lower cost) • Oxamniquine	Use of praziquantel in high-risk populations to prevent morbidity. Improved access to clean water and sanitation.
Soil-transmitted helminthiases	*Ascaris lumbricoides, Trichuris trichiura, Necator americanus* and *Ancylostoma duodenale*	Infectious diseases transmitted by eggs of different species of parasitic worms present in human feces, which contaminate the soil and water in low-sanitation areas. Affects the poorest and most deprived communities.	1.5 billion people infected worldwide.	Albendazole and mebendazole (single-dose oral administration and effectiveness for several months).	Access to clean and safe water, appropriate waste disposal and health education. Periodic administration of anthelminthics to groups of people at risk.

Disease	Causative agent	Main characteristics	Prevalence	Therapy	Prophylaxis
		Wide range of symptoms including diarrhea, abdominal pain, general malaise and weakness. Chronic intestinal blood loss is caused by hookworms.			
Snakebite envenoming	*Venom* (mixture of different toxins)	Life-threatening disease that results from the bite of a venomous snake or snake venom sprayed into the eyes. Local symptoms are pain, edema, erythema, or ecchymosis at the site of the bite or adjacent tissues. Severe systemic effects include hypotension, tachypnea, respiratory distress, tachycardia, altered sensorium and death.	4.5-5.4 million people get bitten by snakes annually.	Aggressive supportive care and sometimes the administration of antivenom.	Snake bite prevention gear such as wearing protective footwear, avoiding areas where snakes live and not handling them.
Taeniasis/Cysticercosis	*Taenia solium* (adult stage: taeniasis / larval stage: Cysticercosis)	Parasitic and generally asymptomatic disease caused by the ingestion of pork contaminated with the tapeworm; however, cysticercosis occurs as a result of the accidental ingestion of the tapeworm eggs in contaminated water and food. Neurocysticercosis is the most common infection of the central nervous system.Symptoms may include severe headaches, dizziness, seizures, dementia, brain lesions, blindness, hydrocephalus, paraplegia, meningitis, intracranial hypertension and even death.	Between 40 and 60 million people are infected.	Oral administration of praziquantel or niclosamide.	Not eating poorly cooked pork, improved personal hygiene, use of hygienic latrines, preventing pigs from becoming infected.

Table 1. (Continued)

Disease	Causative agent	Main characteristics	Prevalence	Therapy	Prophylaxis
Trachoma	*Chlamydia trachomatis*, serotypes (serovars) A, B and C	Chronic infective condition of the eye that gives rise to roughness in the inner surface of the eyelids. Prevalent in the poor communities of sub-Saharan Africa, Asia, South America and the Middle East. It is the cause of blindness or visual impairment in over 1.9 million people worldwide. The bacterium is transmitted mostly among children by close contact and contaminated fingers and clothing; it is believed that flies could be transmitters of the disease.	146 million people with active trachoma.	• Single-dose oral azithromycin • Topical tetracycline • Surgery to treat the blinding stage of the disease	Environmental sanitary measures such as fly control using insecticide spray, health education programs, latrine use and increased facial cleanliness.
Yaws (Endemic treponematoses)	*Treponema pallidum* subsp. *pertenue*	Disabling skin condition and one of the three endemic non-venereal treponemal diseases in West Africa, Southeast Asia and the Pacific. It affects the skin, bone and cartilage of children living in poor and remote communities. Transmission is through person-to-.person direct contact of minor injuries. Infection can lead to chronic disfigurement and disability if left untreated.	59,000 cases reported in 2016 (75% are children under 15 years of age).	• Single-dose oral azithromycin • Single-dose intramuscular benzathine penicillin	Total community treatment in endemic regions.

- A strong commitment between pharmaceutical companies and governments, or international agencies to make prices of new technologies more accessible.

Finally, designing and implementing nanotechnologies at reasonable costs and making them affordable to people in developing countries are key ethical and scientific challenges. This would probably allow to transform a chronic and even fatal disease into a highly curable one, for all patients regardless of their socioeconomic status.

Nanotechnology and Nanomedicines

Almost 60 years ago, the Nobel Laureate in Physics, Richard Feynman with his lecture "There's Plenty of Room at the Bottom," boosted the history of nanotechnology 30 years later [41]. Nowadays, nanotechnology is considered one of the most revolutionary fields of all times and has become a significant matter of importance for some governments in terms of publications, patents and investment.

In this regard, nanomedicine has emerged as a result of the application of nanotechnology in the administration and delivery of drugs or medical devices for diagnostic, therapeutic and preventive purposes. This new branch of medicine employs nanoscale materials (or nanomaterials) and has brought significant advances in the clinical field [42]. In the particular case of nanomedicine, materials with dimensions up to 1 μm are usually considered nanomaterials [43]. These nanoparticles may improve some of the technological issues shown by about half of the approved active pharmaceutical ingredients, such as solubility, cellular uptake, pharmacokinetic and biodistribution profiles, circulation times and clearance mechanisms [44]. Moreover, they may be also functionalized with different moieties, in order to produce a therapeutic effect in a specific target organ/cell, thus giving concrete form to the concept of "magic bullets" introduced by Paul Ehrlich about a century ago, with a better toxicity profile [45, 46].

For instance, the effective treatment of intracellular infections, such as those occurring in the lung, including TB, histoplasmosis, atypical pneumonia, requires a therapeutic formulation that can be easily internalized by alveolar macrophages. For this purpose, active targeting of the nanocarriers to the mannose receptors present in the cell surface of macrophages can be achieved by anchoring mannose residues onto the carrier surface. Other ligands for macrophage targeting can include galactomannan, maleylated bovine serum albumin, O-steroyl amylopectin, O-palmitoylmannan, p-aminophenyl-mannopyranoside, O-palmitoylpullulan, the tetrapeptide tufsin and the surfactant proteins SP-A and SP-D [47, 48]. A similar approach can be achieved for drug targeting to the central nervous system (CNS) using the shuttle angiopep-2 [49]. It is also feasible to target the nanocarrier to surface receptors of microorganisms to further enhance their therapeutic efficacy (e.g., lectin-decorated nanocarriers) [47]. In addition to using surface ligands, targeting of drugs to specific cells can be achieved by tailoring the physicochemical properties of the carriers such as size, hydrophilicity, composition and surface charge [50].

Since the approval of the first nanomedicine, Adagen™ almost 30 years ago, around 70 nanomedicine products have been approved by the FDA and the European Medicines Agency (EMA) for marketing, and double this number are available in clinical trials. Of them, only 11 EMA/FDA-approved nanomedicines are available for the treatment of infectious diseases (Table 2).

Every year, new nanomedicines of previously approved drugs enter clinical trials to investigate their improvement with regard to efficacy compared with conventional formulations. However, most nanomedicines approved to date have shown reduced toxicity rather than improved efficacy. A variety of nanoparticle-based drugs have entered the market and are used daily by many patients. Globally marketed nanomedicines are classified as nanocrystals, lipid-based nanoparticles, polymer-based nanoparticles, dendrimer-based nanoparticles, protein-based nanoparticles, and inorganic nanoparticles [51]. Of them, lipid-based nanoparticles and polymer-based nanoparticles are among the nanomedicines most represented in the clinical setting and in the EMA/FDA approval list. Liposomes, SLNs and nanostructured lipid carriers (NLCs) are the most important representatives of lipid-based nanosystems. Liposomes are spherical vesicles created by a lipid bilayer of phospholipids; SLNs consist of a solid lipid core at room and body temperature; and NLCs consist of a core that comprises a liquid lipid phase inside the solid lipid phase [52]. All these lipid nanostructures are more biocompatible if compared to the polymeric or inorganic nanoparticles, and they have an inherent ability, due to their small size and to their lipid nature, to penetrate the blood-brain barrier (BBB) even without any functionalization [52]. This is crucial for those clinical conditions affecting the CNS. One more advantage of these nanostructures compared to the synthetic polymers is the possibility of their production at large scale, and this is one of the reasons why these nanostructures are becoming more attractive as drug delivery systems. Unfortunately, to date, very few of these systems have been commercially available or assessed in clinical trials, and one of the possible reasons for their major drawback lies in their low loading capacity, as will be further discussed in Section 4.

Table 2. EMA/FDA approved nanomedicines for infectious diseases

Tradename (Company)	Active compound	Nanoformulation	Indication	Approval date
AmBisome™ (Gilead Sciences)	Amphotericin B	Lipid-based nanoparticles	Invasive fungal infections (mold and yeast) and leishmaniasis	EMA (1990), FDA (1997)
Epaxal™ (Crucell Berna Biotech)	Inactivated hepatitis A virus vaccine	Nanocrystals	Prevents hepatitis A	EMA (1993)
Abelcet™ (Defiante Farmaceutica)	Amphotericin B	Lipid-based nanoparticles	Invasive fungal infections (mold and yeast) and leishmaniasis	FDA (1995)
Inflexal™ (Crucell Berna Biotech)	Inactivated influenza virus vaccine	Lipid-based nanoparticles	Prevents influenza	EMA (1997)
Visudyne™ (Bausch and Lomb)	Verteporfin	Lipid-based nanoparticles	Ocular histoplasmosis; wet age-related macular degeneration, myopia	EMA (2000), FDA (2000)
PegIntron™ (Merck)	Interferon alpha-2b	Polymer-based nanoparticles	Chronic hepatitis C virus infection	EMA (2000), FDA (2001)
Pegasys™ (Hoffmann- La Roche)	Interferon alpha-2a	Polymer-based nanoparticles	Chronic hepatitis C and hepatitis B virus infection	EMA (2002), FDA (2002)
VivaGel™ BV (Starpharma)	Astrodimer sodium	Dendrimer-based nanoparticles	Anti-infective agent for prevention of recurrent bacterial vaginosis	EMA (2015)
Arikayce™ (Insmed Incorporated)	Amikacin	Lipid-based nanoparticles	*Mycobacterium avium* complex lung disease	FDA (2018)
Pfizer-BioNTech COVID-19 Vaccine COMIRNATY™ (Pfizer Pharmaceuticals)	mRNA vaccine	Lipid-based nanoparticles	Prevents COVID-19	FDA (2021)

Table 2. (Continued)

Tradename (Company)	Active compound	Nanoformulation	Indication	Approval date
Moderna COVID-19 vaccine Spikevax™ (ModernaTX Inc.)	mRNA vaccine	Lipid-based nanoparticles	Prevents COVID-19	FDA (2021)

Until now, most of the nanotechnological developments have been focused on cancer. In this regard, the number of scientific articles describing nanomedicines for cancer is enormous. A search of the terms "therapy" or "treatment" and "nanotechnology" and "cancer" in Pubmed may deliver more than 8,000 results with only 15 FDA-approved products for cancer treatment [51]. In this respect, the number of FDA-approved nanomedicines for cancer therapy account for almost two products every one thousand articles. Conversely, a search for the same terms replacing "cancer" with "infectious diseases" may result in less than 500 articles with nine FDA-approved products for this kind of diseases, thus representing a 10-fold higher rate of FDA-approved products / published scientific articles for infectious diseases versus cancer. Finally, a search using the same terms but replacing "infectious diseases" with "neglected tropical diseases" rendered only 11 results. Therefore, it is clear that researchers should expand their horizons and use nanomedicines in other clinical fields and not only for cancer. In this review, we will give an overview of the recent advances of the different SLN formulations designed as nanoplatforms for the treatment of infectious diseases.

SLNs: Structure, Preparation and Biomedical Applications

SLNs are colloidal drug delivery systems of nanoscopic size (50-1000 nm) made up of solid lipids (high melting fat matrix) that emerged in 1991 to overcome the drawbacks of traditional colloidal nanocarriers, such as emulsions, liposomes and polymeric nanoparticles (e.g., polymer degradation and cytotoxicity, lack of suitable large-scale production method, low stability, drug leakage and fusion, phospholipid degradation, high production cost, sterilization problems) [53].

SLNs are thus a new generation of submicron-sized lipid emulsions where the liquid lipid (oil) has been substituted by a solid lipid, which in turn, gives the nanoparticle greater resistance to physiological and storage adversities, controlled release and greater protection from dispersed active compounds, properties that vary depending on the composition of the nanosystem.

These nano-size colloidal carriers are composed of lipids dispersed in water or in an aqueous surfactant (emulsifier) solution. These lipids share common characteristics such as low melting points and solidity at room and body temperatures.

The lipids used may be triglycerides (Dynasan™ 118/tristearin), partial glycerides (Compritol™ 888 ATO/glycerol dibehenate, Precirol™ ATO 5/glycerol distearate Geleol™/glycerol monostearate), fatty acids (stearic acid, palmitic acid), steroids (cholesterol) and waxes (cetyl palmitate). Using physiological lipids might decrease the danger of acute and chronic toxicity of SLNs. Various emulsifiers and their combination (poloxamer 188/Pluronic™ F68, poloxamer 407/Pluronic™ F127, phosphatidyl choline, soy and egg lecithin, polysorbate (Tween™) 80, dimethyl dioctadecyl ammonium bromide) have been used to stabilize lipid dispersion [53, 54]. The combination of emulsifiers might prevent particle agglomeration more efficiently. The choice of the emulsifier/surfactant also depends on the administration route with a suitable number of surfactants suitable for parenteral administration. Sodium dodecyl sulphate, tyloxapol, sodium oleate, taurocholeate sodium salt, sodium glyocholate and butanol may be used as cosurfactants, whereas gelatin, glucose, mannose, maltose, lactose, sorbitol, mannitol, glycine, polyvinyl alcohol, polyvinyl pyrrolidone may be used as cryoprotectants, thimerosal as preservative, and dipalmitoyl phosphatidyl choline, stearylamine, dicetylphosphate, dimyristoil and phosphatidyl glycerol may be used as charge modifiers [53, 54].

The proper selection of lipids and surfactants as well as the composition of SLNs, approximately 0.1 – 30% w/w for the solid core and 0.5 – 5% w/v for the surfactants, affects their physicochemical properties such as size, polydispersity, surface charge, short- and long-term stability, drug loading and release profile [52, 54].

Since the solid core of SLNs is hydrophobic with a monolayer coating of phospholipids, the drug is usually dispersed or dissolved in the core. Drug release from SLNs depends on matrix type and drug location in the formulation. One of the major reasons for the fast development of SLNs is their ability to incorporate both hydrophilic and lipophilic drugs, including oligonucleotides, peptides and smaller particles such as supermagnetic iron oxide nanoparticles for controlled and targeted drug delivery.

As shown in Table 3, SLNs have many advantages compared to conventional colloidal carriers, such as biocompatibility, long-term stability, low toxicity, large surface area and prolonged drug release [52]. In addition, their fabrication can be easily scaled up at industrial levels, and most of their preparation methods do not require the use of organic solvents which may affect the toxicity of the final product [51].

SLNs can also be functionalized with specifically modified targeting lipids for active targeting of the carried biomolecules to the desired anatomic site. However, the major drawbacks of SLNs are the expulsion of the encapsulated drug, their tendency to gelate, and their low encapsulation efficiency (EE) [55]. The latter results from the internal structure of the lipid core, which during crystallization does not allow the creation of empty spaces, making difficult for a potential encapsulated substance to remain trapped inside the solid phase.

Table 3. Advantages and disadvantages of SLNs as drug delivery systems

Advantages	Disadvantages
• Ability to bypass cells of the reticuloendothelial system and thus spleen and liver filtration due to their nanosize range • High stability to incorporated drugs, preventing them from photochemical, oxidative and chemical degradation • Feasibility to incorporate either hydrophilic or hydrophobic drugs, with reduced chances of drug leakage • Improve solubility and bioavailability of poorly water-soluble drugs • Ease to scale up • Ease to sterilize • Drying by lyophilization is achievable • Several biocompatible and biodegradable biomaterials are used for the preparation of SLNs • Provide opportunities for targeted and controlled release of drugs • Low toxicity • Superior cellular uptake compared to conventional colloidal carriers	• Poor drug loading or encapsulation capacity • High water content (70-90%) of dispersions • Chances of drug expulsion following crystallization or transformation of the solid lipid • Only highly potent low dose hydrophilic drugs can be suitably incorporated in the solid lipid matrix

Aiming at overcoming this issue, Müller et al. [56] proposed a modified version of SLNs, named NLCs, where the structure of the solid lipid core contains imperfections that increase the internal free space of the solid, resulting in higher levels of loaded drug. To achieve this imperfect crystal structure, it is recommended to mix liquid lipids with the solid lipid as well as the use of lipids like mono-, di- and triglycerides with different chain lengths [55]. This next generation of SLNs display improved loading efficiency and better stability and prevent drug expulsion during storage [57]. In the case of hydrophobic drugs, increased loading efficiency is achieved due to the inherent property of some drugs to better dissolve in the liquid than the solid lipid. Based on this fact, an increased solubility of the drug leads to higher loading efficiencies [58].

Moreover, in the case of hydrophilic drugs, a lipid conjugation approach is followed, where the functional group of the drug (e.g., amine group) can be conjugated with the functional group (e.g., carboxylic acid group) of lipids such as oleic acid, through carbodiimide or another type of chemicals [53, 54]. NLCs make use of the same lipids mentioned above for SLNs as well as liquid lipids, such as almond oil, cetiol, corn oil, Mygliol™ 812 N, oleic acid, olive oil, peanut oil, sesame oil, soybean oil, Speziol™ EOL NF, Tegosoft™ M, Tegosoft™ P, Suppocire™ NC, L-phosphatidyl choline (PC), soy lecithin, and Capmul™ MCM C8. The surfactants used for the preparation of NLCs are also similar to those used for SLNs, and include: Cremophor™ EL, Cremophor™ RH, Eumulgin SML, Lutrol F68, Span™ 85, Tego Care 450, Speziol™ TPGS Pharma, Myrj™ 59, Tween™ 20, Tween™ 80, N-[1-(2,3-dioleyloxy) propyl]-N,N,N-trimethyl-ammonium chloride (DOTMA) [52]. The ratio between the solid lipid and the liquid lipid can range from 4:1 to 1:4, the surfactant concentration from 0.25 to 6% (w/v), and the total lipid concentration from 1 to 30% (w/v).

Different methods were described for the preparation of SLNs. Among them, the high-pressure homogenization technique (HPH) is the most popular because of its easy handling its relatively low cost, ability of large-scale production, and capacity to produce nanoparticles with small size and low polydispersity index.

The preparation methods can be divided into: high energy (HPH, ultrasonication, high shear homogenization, and supercritical fluid technique), low energy (microemulsion, double emulsion, phase inversion temperature, and membrane contactor) and based on the organic solvent (emulsification-solvent evaporation, emulsification-solvent diffusion, and solvent injection).

It should be emphasized that the size range and the polydispersity of the particles depend on the amount of energy that is given to the system. Low energies lead to higher polydispersity, larger particles and lower stability. Increasing the amount of energy, the size and polydispersity are reduced, and stability is increased. In certain cases, a combination of these techniques is applied in order to obtain nano-sized particles. The type of solid lipids, liquid lipids and surfactants that are used also affects the final size and polydispersity of SLNs, since steric hindrances due to functional groups or the length of the chain and crystallization parameters are different depending on the materials.

In the case of hydrophilic drugs, a double emulsification method can be used.

For the characterization of SLNs, dynamic light scattering (DLS) is used to determine particle size, polydispersity index (PDI) and zeta potential. Electron microscopy techniques such as scanning electron microscopy (SEM) produce 3D images of the particles, surface morphology, whereas transmission electron microscopy (TEM) provides information about the size and shape of nanoparticles as well as of the internal structure. The degree of crystallinity of lipid particles can be determined with the aid of differential scanning calorimetry (DSC). Powder X-ray diffractometry (PXRD) can be applied for the analysis of the crystal structure of SLNs. Acoustic spectroscopy can also be used to determine the size and surface charge of the nanoparticles.

To learn more, readers are directed to comprehensive reviews that have been published elsewhere [52-54].

Although all of the above-mentioned nanostructures have been used as drug delivery systems for treating and/or preventing infectious diseases, this chapter will focus only on SLNs.

SLNs and Fungal Infections

Fungal diseases are considered a serious matter of health concern worldwide, having a great impact on human morbidity and mortality, especially among immunocompromised individuals such as organ transplant recipients and cancer or HIV/AIDS patients. It is estimated that over 300 million people suffer from serious fungal-related diseases. Of the 1.5 million fungal species that exist worldwide, approximately 300 are capable of producing disease in humans [59]. They can cause superficial infections, primarily in immunocompetent individuals, and opportunistic, invasive, life-threatening infections, primarily in immunosuppressed patients. These diseases range from those that are relatively less serious but at times can be tenacious superficial mycoses of the skin and nails that affect 25% of the population around the world to life-threatening invasive infections that kill 1.5-2 million people per year, which is more than malaria and similar to TB [60].

Despite all the achieved advances in prevention and diagnosis, the incidence of fungal infections is still on the rise, particularly owing to the increase in the number of immunocompromised patients [61].

It is estimated that species from genera *Aspergillus, Candida, Cryptococcus*, and *Pneumocystis* are responsible for more than 90% of all reported fungal-related deaths [62]. In addition, endemic systemic mycoses caused by thermal-dimorphic fungi such as *Blastomyces dermatitidis, Coccidioides immitis, Coccidioides posadasii, H. capsulatum, Paracoccidioides brasiliensis, Paracoccidioides lutzii,* and *Talaromyces marneffei* are responsible for approximately 65,000 life-threatening cases each year worldwide [63]. However, incidence data of all mycoses are usually inaccurate due to underdiagnosis and underreporting.

Current available antifungal agents for the treatment of deep mycoses, invasive fungal infections and systemic mycoses include polyenes (amphotericin B, AmB), triazoles (fluconazole, itraconazole, voriconazole, posaconazole and isavuconazole) and echinocandins (caspofungin, anidulafungin and micafungin) (Table 4).

Polyenes were the first class of antifungal drugs that emerged in the late 1950s. Among, this drug class, AmB is the most used for the treatment of systemic and deep fungal infections and is considered the gold standard for the therapy of most life-threatening fungal diseases due to its fungicidal effect [64].

AmB was first introduced in the market in 1958 as a sodium deoxycholate solution (AmB-SD, Fungizone™) administered by IV route. Its high toxicity, particularly, nephrotoxicity, which is related to self-associated AmB (dimers, oligomers) was then circumvented by the development of lipid formulations [65]. Among them, L-AmB (AmBisome™, a unilamellar liposomal formulation of AmB in which particle diameters are almost 80 nm [66]), AmB lipid complex (Abelcet™, composed of AmB, dimyristoyl phosphateidylcholine and dimyristoyl phosphatidylglycerol in a 1:1 drug-to-lipid ratio that forms ribbon-like complexes of 1.6 to 11 μm [67]) and AmB colloidal dispersion (Amphocil™/Amphotec™, composed of AmB and cholesteryl sulfate at a 1:1 molar ratio that forms stable colloidal discoidal structures with diameters of 100 ± 22 nm [68]). However, all these three lipidic alternatives are more expensive than AmB-SD, limiting its use in public health care systems with scarce resources. For instance, the 50-mg vial of AmB-SD required to administer a typical 0.7-mg/kg dose to a 70-kg adult costs 20 US dollars, whereas the licensed doses of the lipid formulations of AmB, which are 3–6 mg/kg for the same 70-kg adult, cost 10-50 times more.

Table 4. Current available antifungal agents for the treatment of deep mycoses, invasive fungal infections and systemic mycoses

Drug class	Drug (brand name)	FDA approval date	Target	Mechanism of action	Antifungal spectrum	Administration form	Most commonly reported side effects
Polyenes	Amphotericin B sodium deoxycholate solution (Fungizone™)	1966 (currently discontinued)	Ergosterol	Disruption of the fungal cell membrane by binding to ergosterol, oxidative damage and stimulation of pro-inflammatory responses.	Fungicidal activity against *Candidia* spp, *Aspergillus* spp., *Mucorales*, *C. neoformans*, *B. dematitidis*. *C. immitis* and *H. capsulatum*.	Intravenous	Nephrotoxicity, hepatotoxicity and infusion reactions
	Amphotericin B lipid complex (Abelcet™)	1995					
	Amphotericin B colloidal dispersion (Amphotec™)	1996					
	Amphotericin B Liposomal (AmBisome™)	1997					
Triazoles	Fluconazole (Diflucan™)	1990	Cytochrome P450 enzyme sterol 14α-demethylase (CYP51)	Inhibition of the *de novo* biosynthesis of ergosterol.	Activity against *Candida* spp, *Aspergillus* spp., Mucorales, *C. neoformans*, *B. dematitidis*. *C. immitis* and *H. capsulatum*. Invasive and systemic fungal infections.	Oral, intravenous	Hepatotoxicity, gastrointestinal distress and infusion-related reactions
	Itraconazole (Sporanox™)	1992					
	Voriconazole (Vfend™)	2002					
	Posaconazole (Noxafil™)	2006					
	Isavuconazole (Cresemba™)	2015					

Drug class	Drug (brand name)	FDA approval date	Target	Mechanism of action	Antifungal spectrum	Administration form	Most commonly reported side effects
Echinocandins	Caspofungin (Cancidas™)	2001	(1,3)-β-D-glucan synthase	Damage of the fungal wall by inhibiting the enzyme responsible for the synthesis of glucan, a major component of the fungal cell wall.	Fungistatic activity against *Aspergillus* spp. and fungicidal activity against most *Candida* spp.	Intravenous	Hepatotoxicity, gastrointestinal distress and infusion-related reactions
	Micafungin (Mycamine™)	2005					
	Anidulafungin (Eraxis™)	2006					

Triazole class of antifungals are compounds that contain three nitrogen atoms in their azole ring [1-(1,2,4-triazole)]. They are considered one of the most potent antifungal drugs and are the prime focus of many pharmaceutical companies.

First-generation triazoles (fluconazole and itraconazole) showed great promise in the treatment of invasive and systemic fungal infections when they were first introduced in the United States market. Then, a decade later, second-generation triazoles (voriconazole, posaconazole, and isavuconazole) were developed and introduced to the market. They display a better antifungal potency, specificity and a broader spectrum of activity than first-generation precursors [68].

Even though azoles represent the major class of antifungal drugs, each of them still have limitations, such as spectrum of activity, resistance, side effects, drug-drug interactions or pharmacokinetic profile [69]. For instance, many IV formulations require cyclodextrin as excipient to increase solubility and there are no intramuscular administration routes available for any of them [70]. Among azoles, itraconazole is the antifungal of choice for the treatment of mycetoma, chromoblastomycosis and other deep mycoses that are considered NTDs (Table 1).

Echinocandins are cyclic lipopeptide molecules that display fungistatic activity against *Aspergillus* spp., fungicidal activity against most *Candida* spp., including fluconazole-resistant strains, such as *Candida krusei* and no activity against *Scedosporium* spp., *Fusarium* spp. and *Cryptococcus neoformans* [71]. All echinocandins are currently available for IV administration.

Despite all the advances in antifungal therapy for the treatment of deep, invasive and systemic mycoses, limitations related to drug physicochemical properties (i.e., poor aqueous solubility, poor oral bioavailability), toxicity and drug interactions restrict the formulation options and efficacy of several antifungal drugs. Sometimes, patient hospitalization for the administration of antifungals may be required [72]. Additionally, long-term therapies and clinical interventions due to side effects are needed, increasing the economic costs related to fungal diseases. Recently, drug resistance has also become a worrisome issue and life-threatening fungal infections are becoming more difficult to treat [73].

SLNs hold great promise to overcome all the above-mentioned limitations due to their ability to enhance drug aqueous solubility, bioavailability and antifungal efficacy. In addition, drug incorporation into SLNs could greatly reduce their toxicity and might be used for their controlled release.

For instance, Bianco et al. developed an SLN formulation containing AmB that displayed a higher antifungal activity than Fungizone™. Although yeast susceptibility to AmB-loaded SLNs is probably limited by the high drug EE% within the lipid matrix, SLNs increase the inhibiting effect of AmB compared to that of the free drug [74]. Patel & Pravale produced an orally administrable dosage form of AmB by encapsulating this poorly-water soluble drug in SLNs (AmbiOnp) [75]. This novel formulation of AmB alleviated toxicity and improved its oral bioavailability and antifungal activity. In this regard, AmbiOnp displayed a relative bioavailability of 1.05-fold, and a Cmax of 1,109.31 ± 104.79 ng/ml after 24 h compared to the commercial formulation Fungizone™ given by the intravenous route, which reached a Cmax of 1,417.49 ± 85.52 ng/ml [76].

In vivo biodistribution studies reported that renal tissue levels of AmB in the case of AmbiOnp were found to be considerably low at 8 h (84.50 ± 22.896 ng/g) and went undetected post 8 h, establishing the safety of AmbiOnp upon oral administration. Plasma creatinine concentration, a significant marker of renal toxicity- was measured prior to dosing and 72-h postdosing of AmbiOnp and Fungizone™. Results showed that Fungizone™ exhibited almost 2.5-fold elevation in plasma creatinine level whereas the developed AmbiOnp formulation offered enhanced safety with protective effect and showed significant four-fold reduction in plasma creatinine level [76]. The *in vitro* antifungal activity against *C. albicans* was eightfold higher than that of the marketed formulation [76].

Aljaeid et al. developed a miconazole-loaded SLN formulation for oral administration to alleviate the disadvantages associated with commercially available capsules. High bioavailability and antifungal activity were achieved (Cmax of 13.71±2.15 ng/ml compared with a Cmax of 8.72±1.23 ng/ml for marketed capsules, and an AUC of 294±24 ng.h/ml versus 121±15ng.h/ml, respectively for both formulations) [77]. The *in vitro* antifungal activity against *C. albicans* was almost two-fold higher than that of the marketed formulation [77].

With regard to cutaneous/mucocutaneous fungal infections, oral treatments have pronounced adverse effects, making the topical route an alternative to avoid this disadvantage. Moreover, currently available pharmaceutical forms designed for topical application, such as gels and creams, do not demonstrate effective retention of biomolecules in the upper layers of the skin [78]. An interesting approach to optimize the activity of biomolecules in the skin/mucosa is the use of nanosystems for drug delivery, such as SLNs, which displayed advantages such as increased adhesiveness, great occlusive properties and higher biomolecule deposition in stratum corneum when designed for topical application [78]. In this regard, topical formulations of AmB [79], fluconazole [80-83], itraconazole [84], miconazole [85, 86], ketoconazole [87-89], clotrimazole [57, 88, 90, 91], econazole [92], griseofulvin [93, 94] and terbinafine hydrochloride [95, 96] were developed and showed evidence of maintaining or even increasing the antifungal efficiency when drugs were delivered by SLNs, when compared to conventional marketed formulations.

Moazeni et al. prepared SLN formulations of fluconazole to overcome resistant *Candida* isolates to this antifungal drug by hindering drug efflux pumps [80]. According to Moazeni et al., fluconazole-SLNs provide an effective nano-scaled safeguard that protects the drug from being pumped out by transporter proteins. Moreover, the hydrophobic surface of fluconazole-SLNs may allow the drug to enter the yeast cells more efficiently, more easily, and more quickly [80].

This formulation might be used to treat both superficial and systemic fungal infections.

Itraconazole-loaded SLNs [97] and voriconazole-loaded SLNs with sustained controlled release of azoles [98-100] were developed for topical ocular delivery for the treatment of fungal corneal infections. It should be noted that eye drops are commonly used for delivering drugs into the eyes. The major barrier to the bioavailability of topically applied ophthalmic drugs is incomplete absorption due to nasolacrimal drainage. SLNs have the ability to enhance the corneal absorption of biomolecules and improve the ocular bioavailability of both hydrophilic and lipophilic drugs. As mentioned above, SLNs can be sterilized by autoclaving, which is an essential step toward the formulation of ocular preparations [97]. SLN formulations also display an optimum particle size for ophthalmic delivery as the human eye can tolerate particles smaller than 10 μm [101].

Dry powder inhalers (DPIs) containing AmB-loaded SLNs for the prevention of pulmonary aspergillosis were also developed [102]. The pulmonary route of administration has great potential for the local treatment of lung infections.

Table 5 shows some examples of SLNs used for antifungal drug delivery, including their composition, preparation methods and main physicochemical properties of the resulting formulations.

Table 5. Different SLN formulations used for antifungal drug delivery

Antifungal drug	Excipient formulation	Method of preparation	Particle size (nm ± SD)	Entrapment efficiency (wt %± SD)	Advantages	Reference
Itraconazole	Stearic acid, Compritol™ 888, cetyl palmitate, poloxamer 188, sodium taurocholate	Solvent emulsification/ evaporation	250.2 to 546.9	81.21 ± 0.62 to 90.63 ± 0.48	Site-specific vaginal delivery with prolonged muco-retention, high tolerability, and enhanced antifungal efficacy.	Mirza et al. [84]
	Stearic acid, palmitic acid, polyvinyl alcohol	Melt-emulsion sonication and low temperature-solidification	126.7 ± 1.793 to 199 ± 1.229	68.95 to 94.94	Ocular delivery of itraconazole with high corneal permeability and antifungal efficacy.	Mohanty et al. [97]
Fluconazole	Stearic acid, Compritol™ 888 ATO, Lipocire, Precirol™ ATO 5, Tween™ 80	Ultrasonication	84.8 ± 4.2 to 113.1 ± 15.3	89.6 ± 3.97 to 90.6 ± 3.69	Effectiveness of SLNs as alternative delivery systems for fluconazole on fluconazole-resistant Candida isolates.	Moazeni et al. [80]
	Compritol™ 888 ATO, Pluronic F68, L-α- egg phosphatidylcholine	Solvent diffusion	178.9 ± 3.8	53.9±3.23 to 75.7±4.94	Provide long-term therapeutic concentrations at the site of infection for eradication of the fungal burden, improve skin tolerability and proved to be effective in topical delivery of FLZ.	Gupta et al. [81, 82]
	Cremophor RH 40™, poloxamer 407, Carbapol 934, Compritol™ 888 ATO, Pricerol™ ATO5	High shear homogenization/ ultrasonication	292 ± 0.79 to 500 ± 0.26	55.48 ± 1.21 to 82.94 ± 1.24	Superior clinical efficacy of topical FLZ-SLNs gels in contrast to marketed product Candistan™ in treating pityriasis versicolor. FLZ-SLNs also exhibited improved skin penetration.	El-Housiny et al. [83]

Table 5. (Continued)

Antifungal drug	Excipient formulation	Method of preparation	Particle size (nm ± SD)	Entrapment efficiency (wt %± SD)	Advantages	Reference
Miconazole	Precirol™ ATO 5, Compritol™ 888 ATO, Gelucire™, Labrasol™, cholesteryl stearate, poloxamer 188, lecithin Lecinol, Cremophor RH40, dicetylphosphate	Hot homogenization/ ultrasonication	23	90.2	Enhanced oral bioavailability and antifungal activity.	Aljaeid & Hosny [77]
	Tristearin, soy lecithin, Tween™ 80, Carbopol 940	Solvent injection	198.42±11.48 to 425.58±10.5	83.68±2.82 to 92.81±2.46	Sustained release of miconazole. Greater drug deposition into skin and better *in vivo* antifungal efficacy in a rat model.	Jain et al. [84]
	Compritol™ 888 ATO, Precirol™ ATO 5, Emulcire™ 61, Tween™ 80, glyceryl monostearate, propylene glycol, soy lecithin, carbopol 940	High-pressure homogenization	244 ± 3.16 to 766 ± 3.69	68 ± 2.62 to 94 ± 3.60	Topical delivery of miconazole with good stability. Miconazole-SLN formulations could significantly increase the accumulative uptake of the antifungal drug in skin over the marketed gel and showed a significantly enhanced skin targeting effect.	Bhalekar et al. [85]
Clotrimazole	Tween™ 80, Tween™ 20, Pluronic F68, Chremophore™ EL, Compritol™ 888 ATO, Precirol™ ATO 5, Geleol™, Suppocire™ NC, Dynasan™ 114,	Emulsification/ ultrasonication	85.0 ± 1.1 to 178.6 ± 9.1	66.9 ± 3.9 to 87.5 ± 1.4	Sustained/prolonged drug release of clotrimazole for multiple administration routes (topical/oral/parenteral).	Das et al. [57]

Antifungal drug	Excipient formulation	Method of preparation	Particle size (nm ± SD)	Entrapment efficiency (wt %± SD)	Advantages	Reference
	Dynasan™ 118, Imwitor™ 900 K					
	Polyoxyethylene-40 stearate, PEG-40 stearate acryloyl chloride, Tween™ 20, taurodeoxycolic acid, Span-85,Tween™ 85, TMEDA	Microemulsion	202 ± 1.3 to 460 ± 2.1	41 ± 0.09 to 43 ± 0.03	Effective for the treatment of vaginal infections caused by *Candida albicans.*	Cassano et al. [88]
	Dynasan™ 116, tyloxapol,	Hot high-pressure homogenization	~ 200 to 800	~ 60 to 70%	Topical clotrimazole delivery.	Souto et al. [90]
	Compritol™ 888 ATO, Precirol™ ATO 5, Dynasan™ 114, Dynasan™ 118, Tween™ 80, SURFHOPE™ SE COSME, SURFHOPE™ SE PHARMA, DK Ester F 160	Emulsification/ ultrasonication	119±7 to 190 ± 12	75.0 ± 3.0 to 87.5±3.7	Sustained/prolonged drug release of clotrimazole for multiple administration routes (topical/oral/parenteral).	Das et al. [91]

Table 5. (Continued)

Antifungal drug	Excipient formulation	Method of preparation	Particle size (nm ± SD)	Entrapment efficiency (wt %± SD)	Advantages	Reference
Ketoconazole	Trimyristin, soy phosphatidylcholine, Tween™ 80, Carbopol 934, xhantan gum	Hot homogenization	172.2±0.75	92.4±2.5	Sustained release of ketoconazole for topical fungal infections. *In vitro* permeation studies and *in vivo* studies suggested that SLNs can prolong drug release and enhance the therapeutic effect of the drug. Cytotoxicity results showed that solid lipids are physiological and cytocompatible and safe for skin targeting.	Ramasamy et al. [87]
	Polyoxyethylene-40 stearate, PEG-40 stearate acryloyl chloride, Tween™ 20, taurodeoxycolic acid, Span-85, Tween™ 85, TMEDA	Microemulsion	202 ± 1.3 to 460 ± 2.1	33 ± 0.05 to 36 ± 0.06	Effective for the treatment of vaginal infections caused by *Candida albicans.*	Cassano et al. [88]
	Compritol™ 888 ATO, poloxamer 188, sodium deoxycholate	Hot high-pressure homogenization	212.3 ± 7.4 to 214.1 ± 7.2	Not available	Topical formulation of ketoconazole.	Souto & Müller [89]
Griseofulvin	Compritol™ 888 ATO, Tween™ 80, Phospholipon 90 G	Microemulsion	117	66.37±1.93	Topical drug delivery system for griseofulvin with enhanced skin permeation effect.	Aggarwal & Goindi [93]
	RADIASURF 7141, Tween™ 20, Transcutol HP	Microemulsion	165 ± 3.48	Not available	Topical drug delivery system for griseofulvin. Sustained drug release for transdermal application against dermatophytosis.	Anurak et al. [94]

Antifungal drug	Excipient formulation	Method of preparation	Particle size (nm ± SD)	Entrapment efficiency (wt %± SD)	Advantages	Reference
Terbinafine	Compritol™ 888 ATO, Precirol™ ATO 5, Pluronic F127	Solvent injection	274.3 ± 9.49	74.56 ± 1.41	Sustained drug release and skin targeting for the treatment of fungal skin infections. By targeting the drug to the skin, SLNs can reduce the systemic access of the drug, thus reducing systemic side effects. Terbinafine-loaded SLNs are more effective than the commercially available formulation to reduce fungal burden.	Vaghasiya et al. [95]
	Compritol™ 888 ATO, Precirol™ATO 5, Tween™ 80, Cremophor™ EL, RH40, RH60, Gelucire™ 39/01, Gelucire™, Glyceryl monostearate	Microemulsion	80–200	Not available	Topical delivery of terbinafine with improved permeability and decreased dosage frequency (hence improving compliance) and side effects. These optimized SLNs for terbinafine will improve safety, cost, and tolerance of the antifungal therapy.	Chen et al. [96]
Voriconazole	Stearic acid, Tween™ 80, Carbopol 934	Ultrasonication	234 ± 3.52 to 288 ± 4.58	61.91 ± 0.04 to 84.25 ± 0.11	Ocular delivery of voriconazole without causing any significant effect on corneal hydration level.	Khare et al. [98]

Table 5. (Continued)

Antifungal drug	Excipient formulation	Method of preparation	Particle size (nm ± SD)	Entrapment efficiency (wt %± SD)	Advantages	Reference
	Compritol™ 888 ATO, palmitic acid, Pluronic™ F68, soya lecithin, sodium taurocholate, tristearin	Solvent emulsification / evaporation	139.1±2.45 to 334.7±4.11	37.91±2.45 to 64.13±2.94	Ocular delivery of voriconazole with enhanced corneal drug permeation in comparison with the drug suspension. Improved availability of voriconazole in aqueous humor without causing irritation and with minimal systemic reach emphasizing the target delivery attributes of nanoformulations.	Kumar & Sinha [99]
	Carbopol 940, Lecithin and cholesterol	Film hydration	106 to 211 nm	67.20 ± 0.29 to 97.30 ± 0.57	Ocular delivery of voriconazole without causing ocular damage to the cornea, conjunctiva, or iris with better efficacy and antifungal activity compared with the marketed eye-drop formulation. Stability studies showed that the formulation had good stability.	Pandurangan et al. [100]
Econazole	Precirol™ ATO 5, Tween™ 80,	High-shear homogenization	139.6 ± 12.67 to 154.3 ± 4.93	96.5 ± 1.43 to 102.4 ± 3.05	Controlled release of econazole through stratum corneum compared with a conventional gel. *In-vivo* results suggest that SLNs with lower lipid concentration improve the drug penetration rate into upper skin after a short period of application and could be effective for site-specific delivery of drugs to the skin.	Sanna et al. [92]

Antifungal drug	Excipient formulation	Method of preparation	Particle size (nm ± SD)	Entrapment efficiency (wt %± SD)	Advantages	Reference
Amphotericin B	Stearic acid, polyvinyl alcohol 9000-10000 MW	Coacervation	355 ± 17 to 422 ± 51	70 to 100	Increased toxicity towards Saccharomyces cerevisiae *in vitro*, compared to Fungizone.	Bianco et al. [74]
	Sodium taurocholate, EpikuronTM 200, Solutol™ HS 15, Tween™ 80	probe sonication	181.6 ±15.75	95.09% ±1.41	Enhanced oral bioavailability, superior safety profile and improved antifungal activity against C. albicans.	Patel & Pravale [75], Chaudhari et al. [76]
	Compritol™ 888 ATO, Precirol ATO 5, Pluronic™ F 127, Pluronic™ F68, Stearic acid, Tween™ 80	Solvent diffusion	111.1 ± 2.2 to 415.8 ± 4.4	93.8 ± 1.8	Greater skin deposition, lower skin irritation and better anti-fungal activity than conventional gel.	Butani et al. [79]
	Distearoyl phosphatidylglycerol, Soybean lecithin, PEG 400, Tween™ 80, sucrose	Solvent emulsification-evaporation	176.7 ± 5.09 to 393.6 ± 47.5	89.30 ± 3.47	Dry powder inhalers containing amphotericin B-loaded solid lipid nanoparticles for prevention of pulmonary aspergillosis.	Mehrabani et al. [102]

SLNs and Viral Infections

Emerging and reemerging viruses represent a major hazard to human health, as has been illustrated by the recent outbreaks reported in different geographical areas of the world, including the outbreaks caused by CHIKV, DENV, EBOV, MBV, Influenza A virus (IAV), West Nile virus, YFV, ZV, SARS-CoV-1, MERS-CoV, SARS-CoV-2, monkeypox virus and type-2 cVDPV [103-107]. Moreover, some viral infections became important pandemics with high mortality rates, such as the "Spanish flu" caused by IAV H1N1, the HIV/AIDS pandemic, and the COVID-19 pandemic. Unfortunately, there is no cure for numerous viral infections, such as HIV, although some antivirals can control them. For instance, in the case of IAV and hepatitis B virus (HBV) there are both vaccines and antiviral drugs. However, these viruses constantly mutate and antiviral resistance emerges [108].

Antivirals can display two main mechanisms of action, by enhancing the host immune system, or by blocking a specific enzyme (e.g., proteases, polymerases, integrases) or a particular step in the viral replication cycle (i.e., replication, assembly, uncoating, entry, release). Most current antivirals are far from being the expected "magic bullets" described by Paul Ehrlich 120 years ago, since they can cause serious side effects to the host due to their mandatory intracellular parasitic nature that uses the cellular machinery for their replication. As reviewed by De Clercq & Li [109], less than a hundred antivirals are commercially available for the treatment of few viral infections, including those caused by HIV, HBV, HCV, IAV, herpes-simplex virus (HSV), cytomegalovirus (CMV), respiratory syncytial virus, varicella-zoster virus (VZV) and human papillomavirus (Table 6). For several of them, there is no ideal cure, since the complete elimination of the virus from the host is not always possible using the current therapies, as is the case for HIV and HBV, which are virus associated with persistent chronic infections, and for HSV, CMV, VZV which are virus associated with persistent latent infections. In many cases, such as in HIV or HCV therapies, the combination of antiviral therapy can improve the therapeutic response. However, in most viral infections, limitations such as long-lasting therapies, side effects, viral sanctuary sites and compartments, pharmacokinetic profiles such as non-specific drug distribution *in vivo* and difficulties in reaching target organs, cells or subcellular organelles where viruses replicate and accumulate abundantly, may hamper the efficacy of antiviral agents.

Table 6. Current available antiviral agents for the treatment of viral diseases

Drug class	Drug (brand name)	FDA approval date	Target	Mechanism of action	Antiviral spectrum	Administration form	Side effects
5-substituted 2´-deoxyuridine analogues	Idoxuridine (Dendrid™)	1963	Viral DNA polymerase	They are phosphorylated to be activated and inhibit viral and cellular DNA synthesis.	HSV-1	Ophthalmic topical	Eye irritation or pain, redness, itching, stromal or palpebral edema, hypersensitivity reaction, burning, corneal stippling, vascularization, blurred vision, and increased intraocular pressure.
	Trifluridine (Viroptic™)	1980			HSV		
Nucleoside analogues	Entecavir (Baraclude™)	2005	Viral DNA polymerase	Inhibit the activity of HBV DNA polymerase by competing with the natural substrate and causing DNA chain termination.	HBV	Oral	Headache, fatigue, dizziness, nausea, diarrhea, indigestion, vomiting, sleepiness, lactic acidosis, and liver problems.
	Telbivudine (Tyzeka™)	2006					Increased creatine kinase, nausea, diarrhea, fatigue, myalgia, and myopathy.
Pyrophosphate analogues	Foscarnet (Foscavir™)	1991	Viral DNA polymerase	Selective inhibition at the pyrophosphate binding site on virus-specific DNA polymerases.	HCMV, HSV (acyclovir-resistant strains)	Intravenous injection	Nausea, diarrhea, vomiting, headache, pyrexia, anemia, renal impairment, and seizures.

Table 6. (Continued)

Drug class	Drug (brand name)	FDA approval date	Target	Mechanism of action	Antiviral spectrum	Administration form	Side effects
Nucleoside reverse transcriptase inhibitors (NRTIs)	Zidovudine (Retrovir™)	1987	Viral reverse transcriptase	After their phosphorylation to the 5′-triphosphate form, they compete and act as chain terminators to inhibit DNA synthesis (interfere with viral reverse transcription).	HIV	Oral	Reversible peripheral neuropathy, nausea, diarrhea, digestive disorders, headache, rash, anemia, fatigue, leukopenia, and hypersensitivity.
	Didanosine (Videx™)	1991					
	Stavudine (Zerit™)	1994					
	Lamivudine (Epivir™)	1995					
	Abacavir (Ziagen™)	1998					
	Emtricitabine (Emtriva™)	2003					
Non-nucleoside reverse transcriptase inhibitors (NNRTIs)	Nevirapine (Viramune™)	1996	HIV-1 reverse transcriptase	Bind directly to HIV-1 reverse transcriptase, conformation changes to impair catalytic activity and inhibit DNA synthesis.	HIV-1	Oral	Headache, nausea, dizziness, fatigue, rash, insomnia, hypersensitivity, and increased transaminases (Nevirapine).
	Efavirenz (Sustiva™)	1998					
	Etravirine (Intelence™)	2008					
	Rilpivirine (Edurant™)	2011					
	Doravirine (Pifeltro™)	2018					

Drug class	Drug (brand name)	FDA approval date	Target	Mechanism of action	Antiviral spectrum	Administration form	Side effects
Protease inhibitors	Saquinavir (Invirase^{TM})	1995	HIV proteases	Block the active site of HIV protease to prevent cleavage of viral precursor proteins.	HIV-1	Oral	Skin rash, diarrhea, gastrointestinal upset, nausea, vomiting, dizziness, headache, fatigue, and back pain (Indinavir).
	Ritonavir (Norvir^{TM})	1996					
	Indinavir (Crixivan^{TM})	1996			HIV		
	Nelfinavir (Viracept^{TM})	1997					
	Atazanavir (Reyataz^{TM})	2003					
	Fosamprenavir (Lexiva^{TM})	2003					
	Tipranavir (Aptivus^{TM})	2005					
	Darunavir (Prezista^{TM})	2006					
	Simeprevir (Olysio^{TM})	2013	HCV NS3/4A protease	Inhibits the proteolytic activity of HCV NS3/4A protease.	HCV genotype 1		Rash, pruritus, itching, nausea, headache, fatigue, and muscle pain.
Integrase inhibitors	Raltegravir (Isentress^{TM})	2007	HIV integrase	Prevent the integration of viral DNA into host genomic DNA by targeting the catalytic site of HIV integrase.	HIV-1	Oral	Diarrhea, nausea, headache, insomnia, and hypersensitivity.
	Dolutegravir (Tivicay^{TM})	2013					
	Elvitegravir (Vitekta^{TM})	2012					
	Bictegravir (Biktarvi^{TM})	2018					

Table 6. (Continued)

Drug class	Drug (brand name)	FDA approval date	Target	Mechanism of action	Antiviral spectrum	Administration form	Side effects
Entry inhibitors	Docosanol (Abreva^{TM})	2000	Viral envelope	Inhibits binding of viral envelope proteins to cell membrane receptors, thereby preventing viral entry into cells and subsequent viral replication.	HSV	Topic	Headache.
	Enfuvirtide (Fuzeon^{TM})	2003	HIV-1 GP41 subunit of the viral envelope glycoprotein	Blocks HIV GP41 fusion to CD4+ cell membrane.	HIV-1	Subcutaneous injection	Injection site reactions such as itching, swelling, redness, pain or tenderness, hardened skin, and bumps.
	Maraviroc (Selzentry^{TM})	2007	Chemokine receptor CCR5 on the surface of CD4+ cells and macrophages	Blocks GP120-CCR5 interaction to inhibit HIV entry.	RSV	Oral	Cough, pyrexia, upper respiratory tract infections, rash, musculoskeletal symptoms, abdominal pain, and dizziness.
	Palivizumab (Synagis^{TM})	1998	RSV glycoprotein F	Neutralizing and fusion-inhibitory activities against RSV infections.		Intramuscular injection	Pyrexia and rash.

Drug class	Drug (brand name)	FDA approval date	Target	Mechanism of action	Antiviral spectrum	Administration form	Side effects
	Varicella Zoster immune Globulin (VariZIG™)	2012	VZV	Passive immunization.	VZV	Intramuscular injection	Headache and pain at the injection site.
	Ibalizumab-uiyk (Trogarzo™)	2018	Domain 2 of the CD4 receptor	Blocks HIV entry into CD4 cells while preserving normal immunological function. It is the first CD4-directed post-attachment HIV-1 inhibitor and the first humanized monoclonal antibody for the treatment of HIV/AIDS.	HIV	Intravenous injection	Diarrhea, dizziness, nausea and rash.
Acyclic guanosine analogues	Acyclovir (Zovirax™)	2002	Viral DNA polymerase	Target viral DNA polymerase to inhibit viral DNA synthesis.	HSV	Topical	Skin reactions at the application site, angioedema, anaphylaxis, contact dermatitis, and eczema.
	Ganciclovir (Zirgan™)	1989				Ophthalmic topical	Blurred vision, eye irritation, punctate keratitis, and conjunctival hyperemia.
	Valacyclovir (Valtrex™)	1995			HSV, VZV	Oral	Headache, nausea, and abdominal pain.

Table 6. (Continued)

Drug class	Drug (brand name)	FDA approval date	Target	Mechanism of action	Antiviral spectrum	Administration form	Side effects
	Valganciclovir (Valcyte™)	2001			HCMV		Diarrhea, nausea, vomiting, abdominal pain, pyrexia, headache, insomnia, and neutropenia.
	Penciclovir (Denavir™)	1996			HSV	Topical	Application site reactions such as redness, burning, stinging, rash, pain, itching, skin discoloration, or hives.
	Famciclovir (Famvir™)	1994			HSV, VZV	Oral	Headache and nausea.
Acyclic nucleoside phosphonate analogues	Adefovir dipivoxil (Hepsera™)	2002	Viral DNA polymerase	Inhibit the activity of viral DNA polymerase by acting as irreversible chain terminators after their incorporation into the DNA chain.	HBV	Oral	Weakness, headache, pyrexia, nausea, vomiting, diarrhea, and stomach pain.
	Tenofovir disoproxil fumarate (Viread™)	2001	Viral DNA polymerase and reverse transcriptase		HIV, HBV		Dizziness, nausea, diarrhea, depression, insomnia, headache, itching, rash, and pyrexia.
	Tenofovir alafenamide (Vemlidy™)	2016	Viral DNA polymerase and reverse transcriptase		HIV, HBV		Abdominal pain, depression, nausea, vomiting, and vesiculobullous reaction.

Drug class	Drug (brand name)	FDA approval date	Target	Mechanism of action	Antiviral spectrum	Administration form	Side effects
Influenza virus inhibitors	Rimantadine (Flumadine™)	1993	Viral matrix protein 2	Inhibits viral uncoating within the endosomes by blocking the transport of H^+ ions through the matrix 2 protein channels into the interior of viral particles.	Influenza virus A	Oral	Insomnia, dizziness, headache, fatigue, nausea, vomiting, and abdominal pain.
	Zanamivir (Relenza™)	1999	Viral neuraminidase	Inhibit virus aggregation and release from host cells.	Influenza virus A and B	Oral inhalation	Headache, diarrhea, nausea, nasal signs and symptoms, bronchitis, cough, sinusitis, and dizziness.
	Oseltamivir (Tamiflu™)	1999				Oral	Nausea, vomiting, and diarrhea.
	Peramivir (Rapivab™)	2014				Intravenous injection	Diarrhea, constipation, insomnia, and high blood pressure.
	Ribavirin (Copegus™, Rebetol™, Virazole™)	2002, 2003, 1985	Viral RNA polymerase	Inhibits mRNA synthesis by inhibiting the activity of RNA polymerase.	HCV, RSV, hemorrhagic fever, Influenza virus	Oral and oral inhalation	Fatigue, pyrexia, myalgia, headache, nausea, vomiting, diarrhea, and dizziness.

Table 6. (Continued)

Drug class	Drug (brand name)	FDA approval date	Target	Mechanism of action	Antiviral spectrum	Administration form	Side effects
Interferon	Pegylated interferon alfa 2a (Pegasys™)	2002	Antiviral genes and proteins and immune cells for antiviral defense	Interfere with viral replication by stimulating CD8+ and natural killer T cells; and the expression of innate antiviral genes and proteins that block viral replication.	HBV, HCV	Subcutaneous injection	Pyrexia, fatigue, myalgia, flu-like symptoms, and headache.
	Pegylated interferon alfa 2b (PegIntron™)	2001			HCV		Injection site reaction, fatigue, headache, nausea, myalgia, anxiety, pyrexia, neutropenia, anorexia, and vomiting.
Immunostimulants	Imiquimod (Aldara™)	1997	Macrophages	Stimulates cytokine release by macrophages for wart regression and local inflammatory reactions.	HPV-related diseases	Topical	Local skin reactions such as itching, burning, erythema, dryness, edema, induration, excoriation, erosion, ulceration, fatigue, pyrexia, and headache.
	Sinecatechins (Veregen™)	2006	Undetermined	immunomodulator to interfere with HPV-induced pathways. It has anti-oxidative activities.			Local skin and application site reactions such as erythema, pruritus, burning, pain, erosion, edema, and vesicular rash.

Drug class	Drug (brand name)	FDA approval date	Target	Mechanism of action	Antiviral spectrum	Administration form	Side effects
Terminase inhibitor	Letermovir (Prevymis™)	2017	Viral terminase complex	Inhibits the CMV DNA terminase complex.	HCMV	Oral and intravenous injection	Nausea, diarrhea, vomiting, peripheral edema, cough, headache, fatigue, and abdominal pain.

HSV: Herpes simplex virus; VZV: Varicella-zoster virus; HBV: Hepatitis B virus; HIV: Human immunodeficiency virus; HCMV: Human cytomegalovirus; RSV: Respiratory syncytial virus; HCV: Hepatitis C virus; HPV: Human papillomavirus.

SLNs were developed to overcome many of these drawbacks. For instance, acyclovir-loaded SLNs were developed [110, 111] to overcome the pharmacokinetic limitations of the antiviral drug acyclovir, such as poor oral bioavailability (15–30%) and a short elimination half-life of 2.5–3.3 h, which requires a high dose and dosing frequency (5 times a day administration) leading to poor patient compliance and hence reduced therapeutic efficacy. An *in vitro* drug release study of the nanoformulation showed 78% release in 35 h, versus 58% in the marketed formulation [110]. Therefore, acyclovir-loaded SLNs could be effective in sustaining drug release for a prolonged period of time for the treatment of viral infections, particularly HSV and VZV infections, by decreasing the drug dose and maintaining the drug in the systemic circulation for a prolonged period [110, 111]. In addition, this nanoformulation may be a good choice for the improvement of bioavailability [110].

With regard to HIV infection, one of the most important hurdles to eradicate this retrovirus is the cellular reservoirs that protect HIV from immune system responses and antiretroviral drugs. These reservoir sites are categorized as anatomical and include CNS, lymphatic organs and lungs or cells, such as macrophages and CD4+ lymphocytes which equip HIV to replicate in a stable state and be protected against antiretroviral drugs for a long time [112]. Most of these drugs are unable to penetrate into the aforementioned reservoirs and maintain therapeutic concentrations for prolonged periods, which is considered a major factor in the emergence of MDR and, consequently, treatment failure. Additionally, many antiretroviral drugs, such as ritonavir, are substrates of several efflux transporters, such as P-gp (MDR1) and have poor oral bioavailability, leading to limitations in reaching effective concentrations in viral body compartments, including CNS. Additionally, high-dose administrations cause toxicity, poor patient compliance and increase in MDR and healthcare costs. To overcome the aforementioned issues in delivery of antiretrovirals and in some cases CNS targeting, different nanoformulations using SLNs were prepared [112-126]. In this regard, SLNs have shown significant advantages for CNS targeting by by eluding efflux pumps such as P-gp and endocytosis/phagocytosis due to their lipophilic nature and small size [112-118]. For instance, the SLN formulations of lopinavir, atazanavir and nevirapine have been shown to enhance delivery through the BBB [113, 114, 122].

Furthermore, poor bioavailability and short residence time of antiretroviral drugs can be improved by their incorporation into SLNs as they could increase lymphatic and macrophagic uptake and avoid first pass metabolism [115-117, 119-126]. This will also increase the concentration of drugs at the target site with a lower dose and consequently decrease the adverse effects associated with antiretroviral drugs.

Topical formulations for the prevention of HIV transmission or for the therapy of HSV infections were also developed [127-129]. For the improved ocular delivery of -for example- valacyclovir, a prodrug of acyclovir, a SLN-formulation of valacyclovir was prepared, exhibiting a sustained release profile of >60% in 12 h and an enhanced corneal drug permeation (22.17 ± 1.41 μg/cm^2 h of drug-loaded SLNs *vs* 3.78 ± 1.34 μg/cm^2 h of the drug solution) without causing local irritation [130]. The *in vivo* study confirmed improved ocular bioavailability of valacyclovir from SLNs (AUC_{0-12}: 856.47 ± 7.86 μg h/ml) in contrast to the drug solution (AUC_{0-12}: 470.75 ± 8.91 μg h/ml) [130].

In order to enhance the antiviral activity of adefovir dipivoxil against HBV, a SLN formulation containing this antiviral drug was prepared [131]. Compared with free ADV in solution, ADV loaded in SLN enhanced the inhibitory effect not only on HBV DNA replication but also on HBV antigen expression. This is probably because the ADV-loaded SLN may improve the cellular uptake of the drug and drug accumulation in the target region through the controlled release profile of drug-loaded SLNs, which served as a drug-container releasing the drug continuously, thus enhancing the drug effect [131].

In an attempt to increase the oral bioavailability of the IAV inhibitor zanamivir (almost 2%), several nanotechnological approaches were described, including SLNs [132, 133].

To overcome the poor performance of ganciclovir against encephalitis caused by CMV, which is related to its inability to efficiently cross the BBB, Ren et al. prepared borneol-modified ganciclovir-loaded SLNs as a promising approach [134]. Borneol, a monoterpenoid component of medicinal plants, which enhances the distribution of drugs in the brain by increasing BBB permeability, was able to enhance the transport of ganciclovir incorporated into SLNs to the brain in mice after their intravenous administration [134].

Table 7 shows some examples of the SLNs used for antiviral drugs, including their polymeric composition, preparation methods and main physicochemical properties of the resulting formulations.

Table 7. Different SLN formulations used for antiviral drug delivery

Antiviral drug	Excipient formulation	Method of preparation	Particle size (nm ± SD)	Entrapment efficiency (wt % ± SD)	Advantages	References
Acyclovir	Stearic acid, Epikuron 200, sodium taurocholate	Emulsification and low- temperature solidification method	180 ± 1.2	78	Acyclovir-loaded SLNs could be effective in sustaining drug release for a prolonged period. This nanoformulation may be a good choice for the improvement of bioavailability and reduction in toxicity with good, sustained release over a long period of time.	Parthiban et al. [110]
	Stearic acid, Compritol™ 888 ATO, Tween 80, Pluronic F68, L-alpha lecithin, sodium deoxycholate	Oil-in-water (o/w) microemulsion	172.2 ± 1.32 to 542.1 ± 0.85	56.30 ± 3.25 to 80.57 ± 0.22	Sustained release pattern and good physical stability. An alternative drug delivery system for acyclovir to enhance its bioavailability and therapeutic response.	El-Gizawi et al. [111]
	Compritol 888 ATO, Soy lecithin	W/O/W double emulsion	234±25 to 678±46	31.67±3.51 to 64.18±4.49	Improved dermal delivery of antiviral agent(s) for the treatment of topical herpes simplex infection in comparison to commercially available acyclovir.	Jain et al. [129]

Antiviral drug	Excipient formulation	Method of preparation	Particle size (nm ± SD)	Entrapment efficiency (wt % ± SD)	Advantages	References
Penciclovir	Poloxamer 188, Brij 78, egg-phosphatidylcholine, glyceryl monostearate, Tween 80, Tween 2C	Double (W/O/W) emulsion	254.9 ± 8.2	92.40 ± 1.4	Topical delivery and skin targeting of penciclovir, with a two-fold penetration enhancement through skin in comparison to the marketed cream. In addition, the amount of penciclovir penetration into the dermis from SLNs increased by 130% in comparison to the marketed cream.	Lv et al. [128]
Vlascyclovir	Compritol 888 ATO, stearic acid, palmitic acid, glycerol monostearate, tristearin, Poloxamer 188 and sodium taurocholate	Solvent emulsification/ evaporation	202.5 ± 2.56 to 431.7 ± 2.45	28.01 ± 1.89 to 58.82 ±2.45	Ocular delivery of valacyclovir. The submicron size, good stability, acceptable pH range, higher entrapment efficiency and ameliorated corneal permeation fulfil the prerequisites for an optimized ocular formulation. The *in vitro* irritancy study confirmed the non-irritating attributes of the nanoformulation.	Kumar & Sinha [130]

Table 7. (Continued)

Antiviral drug	Excipient formulation	Method of preparation	Particle size (nm ± SD)	Entrapment efficiency (wt % ± SD)	Advantages	References
					Furthermore, the higher distribution/content of drug in the aqueous humor (in comparison to plasma) suggested higher efficacy of the nanoformulation with reduced systemic adverse effects.	
Ritonavir	Glyceryl monostearate, Soy lecithin, Tween 80, Poloxamer 188	Solvent emulsification evaporation and double emulsion (W1/O/W2)	178.7 ± 4.5 to 254.3 ± 16.6	21.44 ± 6.8 to 53.28 ±12.8	Encapsulated ritonavir in SLNs efficiently maintains its antiviral activity and modulates drug release.	Javan et al. [112]
Adefovir dipivoxil	Monostearin, poloxamer 188	Solvent diffusion	389.4±166.5	15.32±2.58	Enhanced anti-HBV activity as a result of an increased internalization of the drug into cells after drug incorporation into SLNs, due to lipid membrane affinity of the material and nanometer particle size.	Zhang et al. [131]
Lopinavir	Compritol 888 ATO, Pluronic F 127	Hot homogenization/ ultrasonication	90.59 ± 4.26 to 273.1 ± 9.4	93.10 to 99.41	Enhanced drug delivery through blood-brain barrier.	Alex et al. [113]

Antiviral drug	Excipient formulation	Method of preparation	Particle size (nm ± SD)	Entrapment efficiency (wt % ± SD)	Advantages	References
	Compritol 888 ATO, Poloxamer P188 and P407, PEG4000	Hot self-nanoemulsification	214.5 ± 4.07	81.6 ± 2.3	A 3.56-fold increase in oral bioavailability was observed for lopinavir-loaded SLNs due to higher lymphatic uptake in comparison to the oral dispersion of lopinavir in 2 % w/v methyl cellulose. SLNs were able to bypass both P-gp efflux transport and CYP450 3A-mediated hepatic metabolism of the antiretroviral drug.	Negi et al. [115]
Atazanavir	Stearic acid, Pluronic F68	Microemulsion	167±8.3 to 224.5±7.7	89.3+2.7 to 98.9+0.8	Enhanced drug delivery through blood-brain barrier.	Chattopadhyay et al. [114]
Tenofovir	Softisan 100, bovine serum albumin, poly (L-lysine hydrochloride), poly (acrylic acid), low-molecular-weight heparin	Phase-inversion	153.66 ± 11.33 to 378 ± 12.3	8.3 ± 0.7	Vaginal delivery of tenofovir for HIV prevention.	Alukda et al. [127]

Table 7. (Continued)

Antiviral drug	Excipient formulation	Method of preparation	Particle size (nm ± SD)	Entrapment efficiency (wt % ± SD)	Advantages	References
Efavirenz	Glyceryl monostearate, stearic acid, Tween 80, Compritol ATO 888, Precirol	Microemulsion	124.5 ± 3.2 to 362 ± 1.2	46.28 ± 1.05 to 86 ± 1.03	In vitro drug release study has shown 60.6–98.22% drug release in 24 h by various SLN formulations. Optimized SLNs have shown good stability at 40°C ± 2°C and 75 ± 5% relative humidity for 180 days. Efavirenz- loaded SLNs exhibited almost 5.32-fold increase in peak plasma concentration (C max) and 10.98-fold increase in AUC in comparison to Efavirenz suspension.	Gaur et al. [116]
	Compritol 888 ATO (glyceryl behenate), Gelucire 44/14, Poloxamer 188, soy lecithin	Hot homogenization /ultrasonication	160.12±5.20	85.6	Enhanced oral bioavailability and targeting of efavirenz to oral lymphatic region.	Makwana et al. [125]
	Glyceryl tripalmitate (tripalmitin), glyceryl monostearate, glyceryl tristearate, poloxamers Pluronic F68 and Pluronic F127), Compritol™ 888 ATO	High-pressure homogenization	566.4 ± 7.4 to 891.1 ± 8.1	16.50 ± 0.51 to 23.93 ± 0.31	*In-vivo* pharmacokinetic studies revealed increased concentration of the drug in the brain, as desired, when administered through intranasal route.	Gupta et al. [126]

Antiviral drug	Excipient formulation	Method of preparation	Particle size (nm ± SD)	Entrapment efficiency (wt % ± SD)	Advantages	References
Zidovudine	Stearic acid, polyvinyl alcohol, Aloe Vera,	Double emulsion solvent evaporation	222±2.6 to 434±2.7	47.7 ± 2.2 to 88.12 ± 2.1	The modification of SLNs with Aloe Vera resulted in favorable drug loading and release profiles as well as good cellular interaction compared to the unmodified SLNs. *In vitro* cellular uptake efficiency of modified nanoparticles could be suitable for delivering zidovudine to brain cells.	Joshy et al. [117]
	Tripalmitin, tristearin, trilaurin, trimyristin, Tween 80, polyvinyl alcohol	W/O/W double emulsion solvent evaporation	620 ± 24 to 905 ± 13	15.65 ± 1.49 to 27.34 ± 0.42	Successful entrapment of a hydrophilic drug within a lipid core and stability for three months.	Singh et al. [119]
Zidovudine and Lamivudine	Stearic acid, cocoa butter, glyceryl monostearate, Lecithin, Castor oil, Tween 80, Poloxamer 188	High shear homogenization and solvent evaporation	417.973 ± 0.41 to 763.798 ± 0.48	89.1 to 98.7	SLNs showed higher drug concentrations in reticuloendothelial system organs than in polymeric nanoparticles. Therefore, SLNs were selectively taken up by macrophages, aiding in the effective targeting of these drugs in AIDS/HIV treatment.	Sankar et al. [120]

Table 7. (Continued)

Antiviral drug	Excipient formulation	Method of preparation	Particle size (nm ± SD)	Entrapment efficiency (wt % ± SD)	Advantages	References
Stavudine	Dynasan 114 (Trimyristin), Solutol HS 15, Plurol® Oleique CC 497, Poloxamer 188	High-pressure homogenization	75 ± 1.22	Not available	Active delivery of stavudine-loaded SLNs to lymphatic tissues.	Shegokar & Sink [121]
Saquinavir	Cocoa butter, cholesterol, stearylamine, Tween 80, Esterquat 1	Solvent diffusion	~ 300	Not available	Brain-targeting delivery of saquinavir.	Kuo & Wang [118]
Nevirapine	Kokum butter, Pluronic F68, glyceryl monostearate, Tween 80	Nanoprecipitation	177.80 ± 0.82	31.87±0.42	Brain-targeting delivery of nevirapine.	Lahkar & Kumar [122]
Darunavir	Compritol™ 888 ATO, Precirol™ ATO 5, Dynasan™ 116, hydrogenated castor oil, Poloxamer 188, sodium oleate, polyvinyl alcohol	High-pressure homogenization	99 ± 1.14 to 181 ± 1.16	42.25 ± 3.12 to 91.4 ± 2.42	*In-vivo* pharmacokinetic studies in rats showed a significant increase in oral bioavailability of darunavir-loaded SLNs in comparison to plain drug suspension and reference tablets.	Deasai et al. [123]
Didanosine	Stearic acid, glyceryl tripalmitate, yellow beeswax, theobroma oil, glycerol monostearate, sodium lauryl sulfate, Poloxamer 188, Tween 80, Span 85,	Hot homogenization/ ultrasonication	159.0 ± 1.3 to 332.7 ± 93.1	1.55 ± 3.00 to 14.48 ± 2.60	Buccal delivery of didanosine.	Jones et al. [124]

Antiviral drug	Excipient formulation	Method of preparation	Particle size (nm ± SD)	Entrapment efficiency (wt % ± SD)	Advantages	References
	Solutol HS 15, sodium deoxycholate, triethyl citrate, mucin, Compritol 888 ATO, Crodamol MM, Crodamol CP, Eudragit RS 100					
Zanamivir	Glycerol monostearate, Compritol™ 888 ATO, Precirol™ ATO, soybean lecithin, Poloxamer 188, polyvinyl alcohol	Double emulsion (W/O/W) solvent evaporation	224.9±45.1 to 324.2±12.6	42.4±7.1 to 55.7±3.8	Sustained release of zanamivir-loaded SLNs. However, compared to zanamivir solution, zanamivir-loaded SLNs showed a significant decrease in drug penetration across Caco-2 cell monolayers, an *in vitro* model for intestinal permeability.	Shi et al. [132]
	Glyceryl monostearate, egg-phosphatidylcholine, poloxamer 188	Double emulsion (W/O/W) solvent evaporation	183.9	36.1	*In vitro* release studies of SLNs using phosphate buffer solution (pH 6.8), showed over 70% release at 4 h.	Cao et al. [133]

Table 7. (Continued)

Antiviral drug	Excipient formulation	Method of preparation	Particle size (nm ± SD)	Entrapment efficiency (wt % ± SD)	Advantages	References
Ganciclovir	Borneol, glyceryl monostearate, soy lecithin, polyoxyethylene glycol palmitostearate, Poloxamer 188, Cremophor ELP	Microemulsion	113.7 ± 5.5 to 142.5 ± 6.3	62.76 ± 2.04 to 67.68 ± 2.80	Borneol-modified SLNs enhanced the distribution of ganciclovir to brain compared with a commercial ganciclovir injection and SLNs without borneol modification.	Ren et al. [134]

SLNs and Parasitic Infections

Parasitic infections are caused by pluricellular eukaryotes named helminths (cestodes, nematodes and trematodes) or by unicellular eukaryotes named protozoans (phyla Sarcodina, Mastigophora, Apicomplexa and Ciliophora contain the most important species causing human disease). They often produce high burdens of disease in low- and middle-income countries, particularly in both the tropics and subtropics. However, parasites can also affect people living in developed countries.

Parasitic diseases are frequently transmitted to humans via contaminated food and soils as is the case of helminth diseases and toxoplasmosis [135] or by bites of infected vectors, such as malaria, human African trypanosomiasis, Chagas disease, leishmaniasis, filariasis and schistosomiasis [136]. Among the parasitic infections, malaria causes the highest mortality rates worldwide. Indeed, it is estimated that this protozoan kills approximately 660,000 people each year, most of them young children in sub-Saharan Africa [137]. Additionally, millions of others die from Chagas disease, African trypanosomiasis, strongyloidiasis, amebiasis, leishmaniasis, ascariasis and schistosomiasis [138].

Noteworthy, many parasitic diseases are often considered neglected (Table 1), primarily affecting vulnerable, marginalized and rural populations of low-income countries. Lack of school/work attendance, growth retardation in children, impairment of cognitive skills and development in young children are among the devastating consequences of suffering from NTDs along with the serious economic burden on entire countries [139]. The antiparasitic drugs indicated by the WHO to treat the most prevalent parasitic NTDs are shown in Table 8.

Recent advances in nanotechnology using SLNs have opened a door for enhancing the efficacy of drugs for the therapy of different parasitic diseases.

For instance, with regard to schistosomiasis, a NTD for which the only currently available commercial drug is praziquantel, efficacy was only documented for the adult forms of the parasite, with minimal degree of efficacy against juvenile and immature forms. In addition, MDR against praziquantel has been reported. The fact that this drug passes through the gastrointestinal tract by passive diffusion to quickly reach the bloodstream, undergoing rapid metabolism might account for the insensitivity of juvenile and immature worms to praziquantel in the systemic circulation.

Hence, larger doses or repetitive treatments were recommended for enhancing treatment efficacy, although these treatments might lead to the high frequency of side effects, and the evolution of *Schistosoma* resistance to treatment. Repetitive treatments might also represent a financial burden on developing countries, justifying the search for novel strategies to overcome existing drug drawbacks. Based on these facts, many formulations of praziquantel-loaded SLNs were designed to extend the release profile, overcome the problems of bioavailability and solubility (due to the hydrophobic nature of the drug and the quick first pass metabolism in the liver), reduce toxicity, and improve the anti-schistosomal efficacy of praziquantel, specifically against the immature forms of the worms in the systemic circulation [140-144].

The encapsulation of the anti-helminthic drug albendazole in SLNs enhanced its poor oral bioavailability related to the hydrophobic nature of the drug and its rapid metabolism, as well as overcame the insufficient long-lasting effect of the anti-helminthic which is linked to the failure to achieve complete cures in albendazole-treated populations and reduced drug-related toxicity [145, 146]. Brain-targeting of albendazole using lactic-acid conjugated SLNs for the treatment of neurocysticercosis were also prepared [147]. Results using this system demonstrated that lactic-acid conjugated SLNs could be a promising tool to treat neurocysticercosis effectively by the dual drug delivery of albendazole and prednisolone to the brain.

Since neurocysticercosis is chronic in nature and requires long term therapy, lactic-acid conjugated SLNs not only targeted brain but also offered sustained and prolonged release of these synergistic drugs in which albendazole kills the parasites and prednisolone alleviates inflammation due to deceased parasites in the brain. Hence, this targeted brain delivery was found to be safe and efficacious for the management of neurocysticercosis [147].

Given that conventional oral therapy of lymphatic filariasis drugs is only effective to kill microfilariae in the bloodstream, but is often ineffective to kill adult filarial worms (macrofilariae) in the complex anatomy of the lymphatic system, SLN-based formulations were developed to target the drugs to the lymphatics and to further increase the residence time in the lymphatics [148, 149]. For instance, Permana et al. developed SLN-based dissolving microneedles as an intradermal lymph targeting drug delivery system for the treatment of lymphatic filariasis [148].

Table 8. Current antiparasitic drugs indicated by the WHO to treat the most prevalent parasitic NTDs

Drug class	Drug (brand name)	FDA approval date	Target	Mechanism of action	Antiparasite spectrum	Administration form
Anthelminthics	Albendazole (Albenza™)	1996	Tubulin	Impairment of tubulin polymerization into microtubules.	Activity against the larval forms of *Echinococcus granulosus, E. multilocularis, Gnathostoma spinigerum* and *Taenia solium*	Oral
	Mebendazole (Vermox™)	1974			Activity against *Ascaris lumbricoides* and *Trichuris trichiura*	Oral
	Triclabendazole (Egaten™)	2019			Activity against *Fasciola hepatica* and *F. gigantica*	Oral
	Levamisole (Ergamisol™)	1990 (currently discontinued)	Nicotinic acetylcholine receptors	Activation of nicotinic acetylcholine receptors in muscular cells leading to a reduction in male ability to copulate.	Activity against *A. lumbricoides, Necator americanus and Ancylostoma duodenale*	Oral
	Niclosamide (Niclocide™)	1982 (currently discontinued)	Electron transport chain	Oxidative phosphorylation impaiment.	Activity against *T. solium (adult form), T. saginata, T. asiática, Hymenolepis nana and Diphyllobothrium latum*	Oral

Table 8. (Continued)

Drug class	Drug (brand name)	FDA approval date	Target	Mechanism of action	Antiparasite spectrum	Administration form
	Pyrantel (Antiminth™)	-	Acetylcholine receptors	Produces longstanding acetylcholine receptor activation and thus a depolarization of the neuromuscular junction causing paralysis and death of the parasite.	Activity against *Enterobius vermicularis* and *A. lumbricoides*	Oral
	Praziquantel (Biltricide™)	1982	Voltage-, ligand- and second messenger-gated calcium channels, intracellular calcium release channels and intracellular calcium buffers	Vacuolization and disintegration of the schistosome tegument product of the tetanic contraction of the parasite musculature.	Activity against *Clonorchis sinensis, Opistorchis viverrinin, Schistosoma mansoni, S. haematobium, S. japonicum, S.mekongy, T. solium, T. saginata* and *T. asiática*	Oral
	Diethylcarbamazine (Hetrazan™)	1950 (currently discontinued)	Host and parasite nitric oxide synthase	Alteration of host and parasite arachidonic acid and nitric oxide metabolism leading to activation of the host innate response.	Activity against *Wuchereria bancrofti, Brugia malayi, B. timori* and *Loa-loa*	Oral
	Ivermectin (Stromectol™)	1996	Glutamate-gated chloride ion channels	Binds to glutamate-gated chloride ion channels of nerve and muscle cells, leading to hyper-polarization of the cells and producing paralysis and death of the parasite.	Activity against *Onchocerca volvulus* (microfilariae) and *Strongyloides stercoralis* (intestinal stages)	Oral

Drug class	Drug (brand name)	FDA approval date	Target	Mechanism of action	Antiparasite spectrum	Administration form
	Oxamniquine (Vansil™)	1980 (currently discontinued)	DNA, proteins and other nucleophilic macromolecules	Alkylation of DNA, proteins and other nucleophilic macromolecules.	Activity against *S. mansoni*	Oral
Antiamoebic and antigiardiasis drugs	Diloxanide (Amicline™)	-	Unknown	Unknown	Activity against trophozoites of *Entamoeba histolytica*	Oral
	Metronidazole (Flagyl™)	1963	Unknown	Probably, through free radical production.	Activity against *T. vaginalis, Giardia lamblia* and *E. histolytica*	Intravenous, oral
	Nitazoxanide (Alinia™)	2004	The pyruvate: ferredoxin/flavodoxin oxidoreductase (PFOR) cycle, and different enzymes: quinone oxidoreductase enzyme NQO1, nitroreductase-1, the protein disulphide isomerase, the glutathione-S-tranferase, the Avr-14 gene, encoding for the alpha-type subunit of glutamate-gated chloride ion channel present in nematodes.	Disruption of important energy pathways for survival and proliferation. Induction of lesions in the cell membranes and depolarization of the mitochondrial membrane.	Activity against *Cryptosporium parvum, Giardia lamblia, nematodes*	Oral

Table 8. (Continued)

Drug class	Drug (brand name)	FDA approval date	Target	Mechanism of action	Antiparasite spectrum	Administration form
Antileishmaniasis drugs	Amphotericin B (AmBisome™)	1997	Ergosterol precursors	Disruption of the parasite cell membrane by binding to ergosterol precursors.	Activity against *Leishmania donovani* and *L. infantum* (visceral leishmaniasis)	Intravenous
	Miltefosine (Impavido™)	2014	Lipids and cytochrome c oxidase	Impairment of alkylphospholipid metabolism and biosynthesis of alkyl-anchored glycolipids and glycoproteins and inhibition of cytochrome c oxidase leading to an impairment of the respiratory chain.	Activity against *Leishmania braziliensis, L.guyanensis, L. panamensisdonovani* and *L. infantum*	Oral
	Paromomycin (Catenulin™)	1997	16S Ribosomal RNA	Inhibition of protein synthesis by binding to 16S ribosomal RNA.	Activity against *E. histolytica, Dientamoeba fragilis, G. lamblia*, *L. major, L. braziliensis, L. mexicana* and *L. donovani*	Intramuscular injection, oral, topical
	Sodium stibogluconate (Pentostam™)	-	DNA topoisomerase I	Reduction in ATP and GTP synthesis and inhibition of DNA topoisomerase I leading to inhibition of DNA replication and transcription.	Activity against *Leishmania* spp	Intravenous

Drug class	Drug (brand name)	FDA approval date	Target	Mechanism of action	Antiparasite spectrum	Administration form
	Meglumine antimoniate (Glucantime™)	-	Unknown	Reduction of ATP and GTP synthesis.	Activity against *Leishmania* spp	Intravenous
Antimalarial drugs	Amodiaquine (Camoquin™)	-	Probably, heme polymerase activity	Probably, inhibition of the parasite cell and digestive vacuole preventing the conversion of the toxic heme to hemazoin.	Activity against the erythrocytic form of *Plasmodium falciparum*	Oral
	Artemether + lumefantrine (Coartem™)	2009	Ferriprotoporphyrin IX or ferrous ions	Inhibition of nucleic acid and protein synthesis.	Activity against the erythrocytic form of *Plasmodium falciparum*	Oral
	Artesunate (Artesun™)	-	Probably, heme polymerase activity	Probably, through free radical production.	Activity against the erythrocytic form of *P. falciparum*	Intravenous, oral
	Mefloquine (Lariam™)	1989	Voltage-dependent sodium channels and 80s ribosome	Inhibition of voltage-dependent sodium channels and inhibition of protein synthesis.	Activity against the erythrocytic form of *P. falciparum* and *P. vivax*	Oral
	Chloroquine (Aralen™)	1949	Acidic cytoplasmic vesicles	Inhibition of the parasite cell and digestive vacuole preventing the conversion of the toxic heme to hemazoin.	Activity against the erythrocytic form of *Plasmodium* spp (some *P. falciparum* and *P. vivax* show resistance)	Intravenous, oral

Table 8. (Continued)

Drug class	Drug (brand name)	FDA approval date	Target	Mechanism of action	Antiparasite spectrum	Administration form
	Primaquine (Primaquine™)	1952	-	Generation of H_2O_2 in human liver and bone marrow.	Activity against the intrahepatic form of *P. vivax* and *P. ovale* and against the gametocytes of P*lasmodium* spp	Intravenous, oral
	Dihydroartemisinin + piperaquine (Eurartesim™)	-	Probably, acidic cytoplasmic vesicles and heme polymerase activity	Probably, production of free radicals and inhibition of the parasite cell and digestive vacuole preventing the conversion of the toxic heme to hemazoin.	Activity against the erythrocytic form of *P. falciparum*	Oral
	Doxycycline (Doryx™)	1967	Unknown	Probably, inhibition of the expression of apicoplast genes, thus affecting the development of viable parasites.	Activity against the erythrocytic form of *P. falciparum*	Oral
	Pyronaridine + artesunate (Piramax™)	-	Heme polymerase activity	Inhibition of the parasite cell and digestive vacuole preventing the conversion of the toxic heme to hemazoin, inhibition of glutathione-dependent degradation of hemazoin and production of free radicals.	Activity against the erythrocytic form of *P. falciparum* and *P. vivax*	Oral

Drug class	Drug (brand name)	FDA approval date	Target	Mechanism of action	Antiparasite spectrum	Administration form
	Quinine (Qualaquin™)	2005	Probably, heme polymerase activity	Inhibition of nucleic acid synthesis, protein synthesis, and glycolysis, and inhibition of the conversion of the toxic heme to hemazoin.	Activity against the erythrocytic form of *P. falciparum*	Oral
	Sulfadoxine + pyrimethamine (Fansidar™)	1981 (currently discontinued)	Dihydropteroate synthase and dihydrofolate reductase	Inhibition of folic acid synthesis by competitive inhibition of dihydropteroate synthase and dihydrofolate reductase.	Activity against the erythrocytic form of *P. falciparum*	Oral
Antitoxoplasmosis drugs	Sulfadiazine (Sulfadiazine ™)	1941	Dihydropteroate synthase	Inhibition of folic acid synthesis by competitive inhibition of dihydropteroate synthase.	Activity against *Toxoplasma gondii*	Oral
	Pyrimethamine (Daraprim™)	1953	Dihydrofolate reductase	Inhibition of folic acid synthesis by competitive inhibition of dihydrofolate reductase.	Activity against *Toxoplasma gondii*	Oral
	Sulfamethoxazole + trimethoprim (Bactrim™)	1973	Dihydrofolate reductase	Inhibition of folic acid synthesis by competitive inhibition of dihydropteroate synthase and dihydrofolate reductase.	Activity against *Cystoisospora belli and C. cayetanensis*	Oral

Table 8. (Continued)

Drug class	Drug (brand name)	FDA approval date	Target	Mechanism of action	Antiparasite spectrum	Administration form
Antitrypanosomal drugs	Pentamidine (Pentam™)	1989	rich-AT DNA regions	Inhibition of DNA replication by binding to AT-rich regions of the genome, and disruption of mitochondrial membrane potential.	Activity against *Trypanosoma brucei gambiense* and *Leishmania* spp.	Intravenous, inhalation, oral
	Suramin sodium (Germanin™)	-	Pyruvate kinase and others	Inhibition of glycolytic enzymes, thus, interfering with energy metabolism.	Activity against *T. brucei rhodesiense* and *T. brucei gambiense*	Intravenous
	Eflornithine (Ornidyl™)	1990 (currently discontinued)	Ornithine decarboxylase	Irreversible inhibition of ornithine decarboxylase involved in polyamine biosynthesis, essential for growth and multiplication of parasites.	Activity against *T. brucei gambiense*	Intravenous
	Melarsoprol (Arsobal™)	-	Trypanothione reductase	Probably, competitive inhibition of trypanothione reductase.	Activity against *T. brucei rhodesiense*	Intravenous
	Nifurtimox (Lampit™)	-	Unknown	Reduction of mitochondrial protein abundance.	Activity against *Trypanosoma cruzi*	Oral
	Benznidazole (Abarax™)	2017	Nucleotides	Oxidation of nucleotides leading to potentially lethal double-stranded DNA breaks.	Activity against *Trypanosoma cruzi*	Oral

Table 9. Different SLN formulations used for antiparasitic drug delivery

Antiparasitic drug	Excipient formulation	Method of preparation	Particle size (nm ± SD)	Entrapment efficiency (wt %± SD)	Advantages	References
Praziquantel	Soybean lecithin, cetyl palmitate, Tween™ 20	Supercritical fluid	23.78 ± 4.52	88.37	Appropriate for oral administration, with a modified release profile (i.e., maximum release rates of 3.85% for the free drug *vs* 7.64% for the SLN formulation) and non-toxicity against fibroblasts. High encapsulation efficiency using cetyl palmitate SLNs.	Andrade et al. [140]
	Compritol™ 888 ATO, L-α-lecithin soybean, Pluronic™ F127	Solvent injection co-homogenization	112.9 ± 1.0	71.63 ± 0.3	Long-term stability for the formulations. The *in vitro* drug release study for SLNs showed a cumulative release of 48.08% for the drug within 24 h, with a similar release profile for SLN suspension after 120 days. *In vitro* cell viability and *in vivo* toxicity evaluation showed that the formulation was safe. In *S. mansoni*-infected mice, a single (250 mg/kg) oral dose of SLNs greatly improved the antischistosomal efficacy of praziquantel both two and four weeks post-infection, demonstrating the efficacy of the novel formulation using SLNs.	Adekiya et al. [141]

Table 9. (Continued)

Antiparasitic drug	Excipient formulation	Method of preparation	Particle size (nm ± SD)	Entrapment efficiency (wt %± SD)	Advantages	References
	Plurol^{TM} oleique, Labrafril^{TM}, Lauroglycol^{TM} 90, Labrasol^{TM}	Hot homogenization	87.32 ± 5.19 to 302.3 ± 5.27	3.02 ± 0.11 to 109.21 ± 2.83	Enhanced praziquantel bioavailability and antischistosomal efficacy with a safe profile despite prolonged residence in the systemic circulation.	Radwan et al. [142]
	Compritol^{TM} 888 ATO, butyl acetate, poloxamer 188, sodium stearate, soybean lecithin	Ultrasonic dispersion	110 ± 19	79.3 ± 0.69	Burst release at the initial stage and subsequent sustained release. Enhanced oral bioavailability.	Xie et al. [143]
	Hydrogenated castor oil, polyvinyl alcohol	Hot homogenization and ultrasonication	344.0±15.1	62.17 ±6.53	*In vitro* release of praziquantel-loaded SLNs exhibited initial burst release followed by sustained release. SLN increased the bioavailability of praziquantel by 14.9-, 16.1- and 2.6-fold, and extended the mean residence time of the drug from 7.6, 6.6 and 8.2 to 95.9, 151.6 and 48.2 h after oral, subcutaneous and intramuscular administration, respectively.	Xie et al. [143]
	Stearic acid, poloxamer 188	Oil-in-water microemulsion	505.6 ± 27.2	Not shown	Decrease in intestinal absorption of praziquantel-loaded SLNs compared to the free drug, suggesting that the SLN matrix could act as a reservoir system.	De Souza et al. [144]

Antiparasitic drug	Excipient formulation	Method of preparation	Particle size (nm ± SD)	Entrapment efficiency (wt %± SD)	Advantages	References
					In a culture of *S. mansoni*, SLNs were more effective than the free drug, leading to the death of the parasites in less time. SLNs displayed decreased toxicity in HepG2 cells in comparison to the free drug.	
Albendazole	Compritol™ 888 ATO, Tween 80, polyvinyl alcohol	Microemulsion	< 40	94%	Higher protoscolicidal properties than the free form of this drug.	Aminpour et al. [145]
	Compritol™ 888 ATO, Tween 80, polyvinyl alcohol	Microemulsification and high shear homogenization	80.9 ± 8.1	59.14	*In vivo* less renal toxicity than the free drug.	Kohansal et al. [146]
	Stearylamine, tristearin, hydrogenated soy phosphatidylcholine, DL-lactic acid, Tween 80	Solvent injection	100.2±1.1	62.2±0.4	Brain targeting.	Devi et al. [147]
Doxycycline, Diethylcarbamazine Albendazole	Polyvinyl alcohol, sodium lauryl sulfate, stearic acid, poly (vinylpyrrolidone), Geleol™, Precirol™ ATO 5,	Hot emulsification-ultrasonication	< 100	Not shown	Enhanced drug concentrations in the lymph system without increasing their plasma concentrations. This could potentially deliver the drugs efficiently to the bloodstream, where the microfilariae reside, while also targeting drug to the lymph nodes,	Permana et al. [148]

Table 9. (Continued)

Antiparasitic drug	Excipient formulation	Method of preparation	Particle size (nm ± SD)	Entrapment efficiency (wt %± SD)	Advantages	References
	Compritol™ 888 ATO, Pluronic™ F127, Tween™ 80				where filarial nematodes reside in infected patients, leading to an effective treatment of lymphatic filariasis.	
Diethylcarbamazine	Compritol™ 888 ATO, poloxamer 188 and soya lecithin.	Ultrasonication	27.25 ± 3.43 to 179 ± 3.08	68.63 ± 1.53	Drug targeting to the lymphatics and enhancement of the residence time in the lymphatics by avoiding opsonization.	Siram et al. [149]
Niclosamide	Stearic acid, Tween™ 80, PEG400	Microemulsion	204.2 ± 2.2	84.4 ± 0.02	Sustained release (93.21%) of the drug in 12 h. Maximum stability at refrigerated temperature. An *in vivo* pharmacokinetic study showed 2.15-fold increase in niclosamide peak plasma concentration as SLN compared to the commercial product. Results including *in vitro* and *in vivo* release studies of niclosamide confirmed that the SLN system is suitable to improve oral delivery of this drug with increased aqueous solubility, permeability and ultimately bioavailability.	Rehman et al. [150]
Ivermectin	Palmitic acid, polyvinyl alcohol, polyglycerol fatty acid ester	Hot homogenization and ultrasonication	312.8 ± 2.40	98.48 ± 0.052	Dermal delivery of ivermectin for the topical treatment of scabies.	Guo et al. [151]

Antiparasitic drug	Excipient formulation	Method of preparation	Particle size (nm ± SD)	Entrapment efficiency (wt %± SD)	Advantages	References
Arthemeter	Dynasan™ 114 (Trimyristin, glyceryl trimyristate), soybean oil, Tween™ 80, soy lecithin, sodium deoxycholate, stearylamine, poloxamer 188	Thin-film hydration	81 ± 7 to 115 ± 7	97.3 to 97.8	This approach will allow parenteral administration of this drug aimed at treating cerebral malaria, overcoming the short half-life of arthemeter in the body, and its current use in combination with other anti-malarial drugs.	Aditya et al. [152]
Artesunate	Glyceryl monostearate, Tween™ 80, n-butanol	Microemulsion dilution	1109 ± 36.43	51.7	The formulation exhibited a sustained drug release profile, which could prolong the drug residence time in the blood and boost parasite exposure to the drug, hence limiting the development of MDR. The permeability of artesunate was also significantly enhanced and this could improve the rate and extent of absorption of the drug resulting in improved therapeutic efficacy.	Masiiwa et al. [153]
Dihydroartemisinin	Stearic acid, palmitic acid, chitosan low-viscous, polyvinyl alcohol, Tween™ 20, Tween™ 80,	Single-emulsion solvent evaporation	184.2±2.0 to 206.4 ± 1.2	62.3 to 48.5	The sustained drug-release profile observed renders the drug highly efficacious even at reduced dosages and may impact positively on	Omwoyo et al. [154]

Table 9. (Continued)

Antiparasitic drug	Excipient formulation	Method of preparation	Particle size (nm ± SD)	Entrapment efficiency (wt %± SD)	Advantages	References
	dodecyltrimethylammonium bromide, D-lactose monohydrate				dosage frequency and consequently result in better patient compliance and reduction in MDR development.	
Chloroquine	Stearic acid, low viscous chitosan, polyvinyl alcohol, d-lactose monohydrate, sulfanoyl, ethyl acetate, low molecular weight heparin sodium	Double-emulsion solvent evaporation	374.6±7.6	78	Enhanced *in vitro* antiplasmodial activity. Incorporation of heparin to nanoparticles improved stealth capable of bypassing clearance by the reticuloendothelial system, improved targeting of molecules enhancing uptake and accumulation, increased stability and solubility, and provides an inherent anti-malarial activity.	Muga et al. [155]
Primaquine	Stearic acid, chitosan low-viscous, polyvinyl alcohol, D-lactose monohydrate, sulfanoyl, and ethyl acetate, Pluronic^{TM} F127	Double emulsion solvent evaporation	218.2±4.3 to 634.5±7.1	64.1 to 75.2	Prolonged drug-release profile which may positively impact on dosage frequency and consequently result in reduced toxicity. Efficacy evaluation in mice showed that the SLN formulation was 20% more effective compared with the conventional oral dose, highlighting the potential of improving antimalarial efficacy of drugs by nanoformulating them into SLNs.	Omwoyo et al. [156]

Antiparasitic drug	Excipient formulation	Method of preparation	Particle size (nm ± SD)	Entrapment efficiency (wt %± SD)	Advantages	References
Quinine	Hydrogenated soy phosphatidyl choline, distearoylphosphatid ylethanolamine, Cholesterol	Ethanol injection	126.4 ± 2.96	38.4 ± 1.43	Conjugation of SLNs with transferrin significantly enhanced the brain uptake of quinine, which was shown by the recovery of a higher percentage of the dose from the brain following administration of transferrin-conjugated SLNs compared with unconjugated counterparts or drug solution.	Gupta et al. [157]
Paromomycin	Tristearin, soy lecithin, stearyl amine, Tween^{TM} 80, D-mannose	Solvent injection	246 ± 32	Not Available	Mannosylated-SLNs showed higher anti- toxoplasma toxicity in comparison to conventional paromomycin and mannosylation may increase up take of the drug by macrophages. This nanoformulation not only increases efficiency of available commercial drugs, but also decreases their cytotoxicity to host cells.	Khosravi et al. [158]
	Tween^{TM} 80, cholesterol, sodium dodecyl sulfate	High shear homogenization, microemulsion	120	42-46	Acceptable efficacy and safety of the SLN formulation against cutaneous leishmaniasis.	Kharaji et al. [159]

Table 9. (Continued)

Antiparasitic drug	Excipient formulation	Method of preparation	Particle size (nm ± SD)	Entrapment efficiency (wt %± SD)	Advantages	References
					This nanoformulation can increase the penetration of the drug into the macrophages, and the efficient uptake by macrophages could be the probable reason for greater efficacy of this treatment. This nanoformulation also enhanced the anti-*Leishmania* immune response.	
Amphotericin B and Paromomycin	Glyceryl monostearate, soy lecithin, Tween^{TM} 80, PEG 400, 2-hydroxypropyl-β-cyclodextrin (HPCD)	Emulsion/solvent evaporation	164.3 ± 17.6	90.3 ± 0.28 to 95.86 ± 0.10	SLNs of amphotericin B and paromomycin using HPCD as a surface modifier for the enhancement of oral bioavailability in the treatment of visceral leishmaniasis. The prepared nanoformulation showed enhanced efficacy compared to liposomal amphotericin B, in both *in vitro* and *in vivo* by reducing intracellular amastigote growth in *L. donovani*-infected macrophages and hepatic parasite burden in *L. donovani*-infected BALB/c mice model, respectively without causing any toxic side effects.	Parves et al. [160]

Antiparasitic drug	Excipient formulation	Method of preparation	Particle size (nm ± SD)	Entrapment efficiency (wt %± SD)	Advantages	References
Amphotericin B	Pluronic™ F127, vitamin B12, stearic acid, Solutol™ HS 15, Precirol™ ATO 5)	Double emulsion solvent evaporation and thermal sensitive hydrogel	306.66 ± 3.35	97.99 ± 1.6%	Increased oral delivery of amphotericin B. SLNs displayed high mucus permeating ability, which can enhance the oral bioavailability of the drug. Complete internalization within the macrophage cells was demonstrated. In vitro studies showed low cytotoxicity and high chemical stability against digestive enzymes. The mucoadhesive study confirmed the interaction of vitamin B12-coated SLNs with mucin. Finally, anti-leishmanial evaluation against intramacrophage amastigotes showed enhanced efficacy (94%) over conventional amphotericin B (75.5%).	Singh et al. [161]

Results including *in vitro* and *in vivo* release studies of niclosamide confirmed that the SLN system is also suitable to improve oral delivery of the anti-helminthic drug with increased aqueous solubility, permeability and finally, bioavailability [150]. SLNs are also suitable for the topical delivery of drug for the treatment of parasitic skin diseases such as scabies to avoid the systemic side effects of the orally administered antiparasitic drugs [151].

Artemisinin and its derivatives are among the most potent anti-malarial drugs, being active at nanomolar concentration in both chloroquine-sensitive and -resistant Plasmodium falciparum strains. Therefore, artemisinin has been included in the WHO list of essential drugs for the treatment of MDR malaria. However, to overcome some of the drawbacks related to this drug (i.e., short half-life, poor aqueous solubility, low oral bioavailability, risk of degradation in acidic conditions and associated risk of toxicity), SLN formulations of artemisinin and its derivatives were developed [152-154].

Enhanced efficacy of antimalarial drugs by SLN formulations were described for chloroquine and primaquine [154-156]. Brain targeting using transferring-conjugated SLNs were described for the treatment of cerebral malaria, due to the high affinity of transferrin for receptors on brain capillaries [157].

Enhanced efficacy of paromomycin and amphotericin B against protozoa, such as *Toxoplasma gondii* and *Leishmania* sp., using SLN formulations were also described [158-161].

Table 9 shows some examples of the SLNs used for antiparasitic drugs, including their polymeric composition, preparation methods and main physicochemical properties of the resulting formulations.

SLNs and Bacterial Infections

One of the bacterial diseases with the highest disease burden is TB, caused by *Mycobacterium tuberculosis* (Mtb), which kills approximately 1.5 million people a year, mostly in sub-Saharan Africa. Pathogenic bacteria contribute to other globally important diseases, such as pneumonia, which can be caused by bacteria such as *Streptococcus* and *Pseudomonas*, and foodborne illnesses, which can be caused by bacteria such as *Shigella*, *Campylobacter*, and *Salmonella*. Pathogenic bacteria also cause infections such as tetanus, typhoid fever, diphtheria, syphilis, and leprosy. Pathogenic bacteria are also the cause of high infant mortality rates in developing countries. Several gram-negative bacteria are resistant to multiple antibiotics such as *Acinetobacter*,

Pseudomonas and various *Enterobacteriaceae* (including *Klebsiella, Escherichia coli, Serratia*, and *Proteus*), often causing severe infections -and even deaths- such as bloodstream infections and pneumonia.

Other MDR bacteria that cause more common diseases such as gonorrhea and food poisoning due to *Salmonella* and *Staphylococcus aureus* as well as *M. tuberculosis* pose a significant public health threat. In this regard, it is estimated that more than 2.8 million antibiotic-resistant infections occur in the U.S. each year, and more than 35,000 people die as a result. In addition, 223,900 cases of *Clostridioides difficile* occurred in 2017 and at least 12,800 people died.

It is worth stressing that TB eradication becomes more complicated due to the presence of latent Mtb forms that can survive for years. Furthermore, the development of MDR strains of Mtb represents a public health challenge. In 2019, almost 500,000 patients developed rifampicin (RIF)-resistant TB, 78% of whom developed MDR-TB [162]. Ten million new cases and 1.4 million deaths were estimated in 2019 [163]. Thereby, TB stands as the "global greatest killer due to a single infectious agent" according to the WHO statistics [162]. In this framework, the main goals involving nanotechnology and TB are related to drug targeting to the Mtb reservoirs, such as macrophages, the improvement of drug bioavailability, the development of novel nanoformulations for different administration routes and the anti-TB therapy improvement looking for enhanced patient adherence.

Among the different nanotechnological approaches employing first-line anti-TB drugs, oral formulations with RIF-, isoniazide- and pyrazinamide-loaded SLNs were developed to decrease the dosing frequency and improve patient compliance [164, 165], as well as for enhanced drug solubility and oral bioavailability [166]. For macrophage targeting of these anti-TB drugs, SLNs were developed using mannose as a lectin receptor ligand conjugate, thus increasing the therapeutic index of these anti-TB drugs [167, 168]. In addition, these mannosylated SLNs were developed to be administered by inhalatory route, which has particular interest in the controlled release of anti-TB drugs directly in the main organ affected by TB (lungs), thus achieving high local concentrations of the drug in the infected macrophages [167, 168]. Taking into consideration the potential mucoadhesion properties of systems in lung delivery, the preparation of chitosan-coated SLNs was also described [169]. Intranasal delivery is considered a promising alternative to intravenous route for a rapid delivery of therapeutic agents to the blood and brain for treating CNS disorders. SLN formulations for the intranasal route were also prepared, for instance, for the treatment of cerebral TB [171]. SLNs were also a promising tool for the intraocular delivery of antibiotics to the posterior chamber, opening new avenues for the treatment of ocular infections, representing a strategy to overcome MDR [172, 173]. Furthermore, the topical ocular therapy of antibiotics could be more advantageous than its oral counterpart because topical administration could minimize side effects as well as reduce the possibility of producing resistant bacterial strains.

Several SLN formulations for the sustained release of antibiotic drugs aiming at achieving an enhanced oral bioavailability, reducing side effects of the administered drug and enhancing antibacterial activity were prepared [174-182].

Table 10 shows some examples of the SLNs used for antibiotic/anti-TB drugs, including their polymeric composition, preparation methods and main physicochemical properties of the resulting formulations.

In summary, of the twenty diseases considered NTDs by the WHO, SLNs formulations were developed as nanoplatforms for at least one of the drugs recommended by the WHO, for tuberculosis, soil-transmitted helminthiases, leishmaniasis, schistosomiasis, echinococcosis, malaria, lymphatic filariasis and scabies.

SLNs and Vaccines

The history of modern vaccine development began in 1796 when the English physician and scientist Edward Jenner discovered the smallpox vaccine.

Vaccines are considered one of the most important milestones in medicine. In an era of unmet scientific advances in vaccine technologies, the development of new vaccines faces challenges including their high development cost and the slow time lines for vaccine advancement to clinical testing (i.e., an effective and safe vaccine typically takes over a decade to be created and validated), among other complexities. The increased occurrence of emerging and reemerging infections could benefit greatly from rapid vaccine interventions. In this sense, the current COVID-19 pandemic is an unprecedented example of this necessity due to the global impact and spread of the SARS-CoV-2 worldwide. For the first time, vaccines were rolled out in less than a year after the initial outbreak of the disease in Wuhan, China, in 2019.

Table 10. Different SLN formulations used for antibiotic/anti-TB drug delivery

Antibiotic	Excipient formulation	Method of preparation	Particle size (nm ± SD)	Entrapment efficiency (wt %± SD)	Advantages	References
Rifampicin, isoniazid and pyrazinamide	Poloxamer 188, sodium taurocholate, stearic acid, mannitol, glyceryl monostearate (1-stearoyl-rac-glycerol), poloxamer 407, hydroxypropyl cellulose, tristearin, Compritol™ 888 ATO, Precirol™ ATO 5	Microemulsion	162.7 ± 9.21 to 373.6 ± 6.79	61.23 ± 0.261 to 86.40 ± 0.274	Improve the antimycobacterial activity of first-line anti-TB drugs. The in-vitro drug release study demonstrated that the drug release from SLNs was slow in comparison to the marketed formulation and pure drugs. *In vitro* cytotoxicity of the SLNs demonstrated two-fold growth inhibition of *M. marinum* as compared to standard antitubercular drugs.	Katak et al. [164]
	Stearic acid, polyvinyl alcohol	Emulsion solvent diffusion	Not available	41±4 to 51 ± 5	Because of the slow and sustained release of drugs from the SLNs, the mean residence time showed a several-fold increase as compared to free drugs. This resulted in an enhanced area under the curve and relative bioavailability of the three drugs.	Pandey et al. [165]
Rifampicin	Stearylamine. D-(þ)-Mannose, glycerol tripalmitate, Tween™ 80 Phorbol 12-myristate 13-acetate	Hot ultrasonication	252 ± 2	95.5 ± 6.0	Mannosylated-SLNs were developed to improve the drug uptake by the macrophages and to be administered by inhalation, protecting it from pulmonary fluid and increasing its bioavailability.	Vierira et al. [167]

Table 10. (Continued)

Antibiotic	Excipient formulation	Method of preparation	Particle size (nm ± SD)	Entrapment efficiency (wt %± SD)	Advantages	References
	Cetyl palmitate, Tween™ 80, chitosan™ (low molecular weight)	Hot ultrasonication	252 ± 2	91.5 ± 0.9	The coating with chitosan is nontoxic, being this sugar a biodegradable and biocompatible polymer that in the simulated mucus layer of the pulmonary barrier protects from the release of the drug, while increasing the mucoadhesion properties retained promoting a close contact of the SLNs and the absorption site, thus ensuring a more effective absorption following pulmonary administration. Therefore, SLNs coated with chitosan have great potential for the pulmonary delivery of rifampicin with absence of cytotoxicity and higher permeability across alveolar epithelial cells.	Vieira et al. [169]
Isoniazid	Witepsol™ E85 (hydrogenated coco-glycerides) Compritol™ 888 ATO, stearic acid, Tween™ 80, polyvinyl alcohol, coumarin-6, stearylamine, D-(+)-mannose, phorbol 12-myristate 13-acetate (PMA)	Emulsification/ solvent evaporation	452.0 ± 16.1 to 530.5 ± 27.1	34.0 ± 7.8 to 50.2 ± 0.5	Enhanced macrophage uptake. Devoid of toxicity. Inhalatory route.	Costa et al. [168]

Antibiotic	Excipient formulation	Method of preparation	Particle size (nm ± SD)	Entrapment efficiency (wt %± SD)	Advantages	References
	Compritol™ 888 ATO, stearic acid, Tween™ 80, soy lecithin	Microemulsion	48.4	69 ± 0.7	Improved oral bioavailability (6 times) and brain accumulation, after administration of isoniazid-SLNs with respect to the free drug solution at the same dose. Insignificant changes in liver concentration coupled with bypass of first pass metabolism and slow release of isoniazid (60%, in 24 h) indicate low incidence of hepatotoxicity. Isoniazid-loaded SLNs showed a 3-fold higher LD50.	Bhandari & Kaur [166]
Ethambutol	Tween™ 80, Poloxamer 407, Compritol™ 888 ATO	Hot homogenization/ultrasonication	56.52 ± 2.05 to 81.83 ± 3.20	98.16 ± 0.66 to 99.04 ± 0.41	Biocompatibility, non-toxicity and high potential for direct treatment of tuberculosis using the inhalatory route.	Nemati et al. [170]
Streptomycin	Soy lecithin, Compritol™ 888 ATO, Tween™ 80	Nanocolloidal aqueous dispersion	140.1 ± 7.0	54.83 ± 2.1	Biodistribution studies showed 3.15 and 11.0 times higher concentrations in the brain and blood of mice, respectively, on intranasal administration of streptomycin-loaded SLNs in comparison to the free drug. Lower concentrations (3.3 times) in kidneys implicate lower nephrotoxicity.	Kumar et al. [171]

Table 10. (Continued)

Antibiotic	Excipient formulation	Method of preparation	Particle size (nm ± SD)	Entrapment efficiency (wt %± SD)	Advantages	References
					Similarly, 12 and 4 times lower levels of drug in liver and spleen, also indicate lesser accumulation in these reticuloendothelial system organs. Lipophilic enclosure imparted to streptomycin, coupled with small particle size, and its purported ability to inhibit Pgp-efflux due to the presence of Tween™ 80, is considered to be responsible for better bioavailability. This might result in an improved efficacy for the treatment of other clinical forms of tuberculosis including cerebral tuberculosis as indicated by the high relative distribution to the brain in comparison to the free drug.	
Tobramycin	Stearic acid, Epikuron™ 200 (soy phosphatidylcholine 95%), taurocholate sodium salt	O/W microemulsions	80.01 ± 11.10	2.5 ± 0.18	Drug concentration was significantly higher in all ocular tissues after ocular and intravenous administration of the SLN formulation with respect to reference formulations and only SLNS allowed the penetration of the drug into the retina; higher intraphagocytic antibiotic concentrations in polymorphonuclear granulocytes and greater bactericidal activity against intracellular	Chetoni et al. [172]

Antibiotic	Excipient formulation	Method of preparation	Particle size (nm ± SD)	Entrapment efficiency (wt %± SD)	Advantages	References
					Pseudomonas aeruginosa were described.	
Clarithromycin	Stearic acid, glyceryl monostearate, Tween™ 20, Tween™ 80, Span™ 80, sodium lauryl sulphate, PEG 400, propylene glycol, Compritol™ 888 ATO, Gelucire™ 43/01, Precirol™ ATO 5, Geleol™, Transcutol™ P, Monegyl™ T18 Softemul™	High speed stirring /ultrasonication	130 to 413	69.9 to 92.4	Ocular delivery, with higher permeation profiles without causing irritation, enhancing therapy efficacy.	Nair et al. [173]
	Stearic acid, tristearin, Pluronic™ F68, Tween™ 80, polyvinyl alcohol	Emulsification/ solvent evaporation	258 ± 25 to 801 ± 28	46 ± 11 to 84 ± 9	Enhanced systemic availability of the drug after oral administration. Improved efficacy in biofilm eradication formed by *S. aureus* at lower drug concentration. *In vitro* cytotoxicity studies showed the safety of the formulation.	Sharma et al. [174]
Norfloxacin	Stearic acid, polyvinyl alcohol	Hot homogenization and ultrasonication	301± 16.64	92.35± 2.24	Enhanced oral bioavailability and antibacterial activity of the drug.	Dong et al. [175]

Table 10. (Continued)

Antibiotic	Excipient formulation	Method of preparation	Particle size (nm ± SD)	Entrapment efficiency (wt %± SD)	Advantages	References
Azithromycin dihydrate	Stearic acid, Tween™ 20, poloxamer 188, and poloxamer 407	High shear homogenization	143.1 ± 3.91 to 167.2 ± 2.70	69.38 ± 1.78 to 89.79 ± 1.56	Improved solubility and thereby oral bioavailability of the drug.	Bhattacharya & Reddy [176]
Ciprofloxacin	Didecyldimethylammonium bromide (DDAB), Tween™ 80, Softisan™ 100	Quasi-emulsion solvent diffusion and solvent injection	272.0 ± 6.03 to 353.8 ± 19.24	82.9 ± 5.55 to 91.1 ± 5.11	Control release and enhanced antibacterial activity.	Pignatello (2018) [177]
Doxycycline	Span™ 80, stearic acid, poloxamer407, Tween™ 80, Palm oil (hydrogenated)	Double emulsion	299.3	Not available	Rats treated with the SLN formulation significantly decreased *Brucella melitensis* CFUs in their spleen and liver compared to rats treated with free drug. The pathologic results indicate that the improvement trend of spleen and liver tissues in rats treated with the SLN formulation was satisfactory.	Hosseini et al. [178]
	Hydrogenated palm oil (Softisan™ 154), stearic acid, Tween™ 80, Poloxamer407, Span™ 80, soy lecithin	Double emulsion	299 ± 34	94.9 ± 3.2	The SLN formulation significantly decreased the microbial load within macrophages (3.5 log) in comparison with the free drug.	Hosseini et al. [179]
Polymixyn B	Tween™ 20, Span™ 85), cetyl alcohol, sodium alginate, 150–170 Da	High-pressure homogenization	439.5 ± 20.42	82.7 ± 5.5	Enhanced antibacterial activity, even in MDR strains of *P. aeruginosa* and less toxicity compared to the free drug.	Severino et al. [180]

Antibiotic	Excipient formulation	Method of preparation	Particle size (nm ± SD)	Entrapment efficiency (wt %± SD)	Advantages	References
	Crodapearl™ past, behenic acid, crodacol™ C90, crodacol™ CS90, crodamol™ SS, crodacol™ S95, arlacel™ 170, crodamol™ MM, crodamol™ CP. Pluronic® F68	Double emulsion method (w/o/w)	202.5±44.43 to 573.6 ± 74.46	93.67 ± 2.30 95.86 ± 1.75		Severino et al. [181]
Vancomycin	Ellagic acid, Compritol™ 888 ATO, Precirol™ ATO 5, Gelucire™ 44/14, phosphatidylcholine	Solvent evaporation-ultrasonication	164 ± 51.43	35.6 ± 8.1	Decreased vancomycin nephrotoxicity.	Aldawsari et al. [182]

Among the few technologies in research in the last three decades, a new class of vaccines based on RNA technology came to light and showed its efficacy in mitigating the severe forms of the disease. DNA as well as mRNA vaccines represent a promising alternative to the production of conventional vaccines due to their flexibility and rapid manufacturing process.

Nucleic acid-based vaccines compared to conventional vaccines such as killed or attenuated microorganisms, toxoids, polysaccharide conjugates, or protein-based subunits have the potential to overcome this challenge owing to their reproducibility in manufacturing, stability under transport conditions, safety profile, and cost efficiency [183]. These third-generation vaccines or genetic vaccines are based on the introduction of foreign DNA or RNA into host cells. The codified antigens, together with an adjuvant and an appropriate delivery system, are responsible for exerting an adequate immune response that protects against pathogen natural infection. More importantly, their use is not limited to the prophylaxis of infectious diseases, but can also be applied in gene therapy, immunotherapy, autoimmunity, allergy and cancer. In fact, mRNA vaccines were first proposed and researched as therapeutic vaccines to fight cancer and other non-infectious diseases as early as 1989 [184].

The following are some of their main advantages: a) safety, since they do not use live microorganisms and do not integrate into the host cell genome; b) ability to induce both cellular and humoral immune responses; c) the antigens encoded in the plasmids are easily modified to respond rapidly to an outbreak caused by an emerging infectious disease; d) lower cost when produced on a large scale; and e) longer half-life (particularly for DNA vaccines), thus achieving better stability in terms of storage and transport temperature, which makes it possible to avoid the cold chain used in conventional vaccines.

However, nucleic acids display some inherent disadvantages. DNA has low immunogenicity and might integrate into the human genome. RNA is rapidly degraded in physiological media and efficiently excreted by glomerular filtration within less than 10 min [185]. Despite this fact, RNA is still considered the best platform technology for developing vaccines against various diseases, both non-infectious and infectious [185]. *In vitro* transcribed RNA vaccines exhibit efficient antigen expression and self-adjuvancy. Adjuvants are often added to vaccines in order to enhance and prolong the immune response; however, they also have the potential to cause inflammatory side effects [185]. Therefore, RNA vaccines are becoming promising candidates as self-adjuvant vaccines with minimal inflammatory side effects.

The physicochemical nature of RNA displays interesting challenges as a gene-based vaccine tool and shares many of the properties described for DNA vaccines (mechanisms of action, advantages and disadvantages over traditional vaccine manufacturing). However, unlike plasmid DNA vaccines, RNA-based vaccines offer the advantage of a certain degree of simplicity regarding their delivery directly into their site of action, the cytoplasm. Hence, RNA-based vaccines bypass any requirement for DNA or nuclear stages with dependence on cellular transcription machinery and transport of nucleic acids to and from the nucleus. This feature is particularly attractive as a means of eliminating its potential integration into the host chromosome. However, as mentioned above, RNA is relatively labile and is likely to be expensive to manufacture at a commercial scale.

Nonetheles, perhaps the greatest potential of mRNA vaccines lies in their versatility, ease of manipulation and production against infectious diseases; especially those with rapid pandemic-generating potential like SARS-CoV-2.

Indeed, studies of mRNA vaccines against viral diseases such as zika, rabies, influenza and HIV-1 were at different stages of phase I/II studies before the COVID-19 pandemic outbreak [186]. Perhaps the most remarkable of these studies are the Moderna Therapeutics mRNA vaccine clinical trials against the Zika and influenza viruses, based on nucleoside-modified mRNA enveloped in lipid nanoparticles. This vaccine platform enabled the company to effectively develop, manufacture and deliver the mRNA-1273 SARS-CoV-2 vaccine within 45 days after the viral genome was publicly available; clinical testing commenced 66 days after genome publication [187]. This world-breaking record in vaccine development shows the crucial potential that mRNA vaccines have in responding to new epidemics and even pandemics.

Despite the structural and functional differences between DNA and RNA, both molecules are negatively charged and thus can share delivery methods. As mentioned above, the transfection journey of RNA aims at the cytosol whereas DNA needs to enter into the cell nucleus to be effective. However, RNA molecules are more fragile and more likely to degrade than DNA, hence relatively high doses are necessary to achieve the desired effect. The electronegativity of both DNA and RNA biomolecules tends to inhibit them from entering most negatively charged cell membranes and unprotected nucleic acids are rapidly degraded by the nucleases present intracellularly and in plasma. Therefore, many delivery techniques have been developed for the introduction of nucleic acids into cells.

Hence, the proper performance of a DNA/RNA delivery system will depend on its capacity to overcome all the biological barriers that may arise.

To achieve that purpose, it has to be able to protect nucleic acids from its enzymatic degradation, to allow targeting to APCs followed by its cellular uptake, to ensure its escape from the endolysosomal environment, and –in the case of DNA, it should be able to direct DNA to the nucleus for further processing. Viral and non-viral vectors were used as nucleic acid delivery methods, and both of them have their advantages and drawbacks, as reviewed elsewhere [188-190]. Among the main advantages of non-viral vectors are their safety profile, low immunogenicity, easy and large-scale inexpensive production, high reproducibility, and no boundaries in DNA/RNA packaging [191]. However, their low in vivo transfection efficiency [192] makes necessary the development of more effective non-viral designs capable of achieving high transfection efficiency without toxicity. Another advantage of non-viral vectors compared to viral vectors is related to mobility. Even though the mobility of the vector within the in *vivo* system is necessary for the efficient transport and delivery of genes, off-targeted effects were observed with viral vectors due to their potential migration towards a different organ of the target after local administration. This is a matter of concern since it might trigger unexpected and uncontrollable results [193].

Two main classes of non-viral delivery methods have been developed, aiming to overcome virus limitations as vectors. One involves physical force administered on cells for the uptake of naked nucleic acid molecules (microinjection, electroporation, gene gun, sonoporation, magnetofection). The other is based on using nanostructured systems made up of nucleic acids and natural or synthetic biomaterials as carriers [194] forming for instance polyplexes or lipoplexes that might adsorb more effectively to the anionic plasma membrane of mammalian cells via electrostatic interactions. In this regard, the use of nanodelivery systems of different biomaterials and the physicochemical properties necessary for the cellular uptake of biomolecules have become particularly important in recent years. Of them, cationic lipid-based systems are the most representative and the most promising groups of non-viral vectors to be used in DNA/RNA delivery because its lipid nature makes it a biocompatible system to interact with the lipid bilayer of cell membranes, promoting cellular entry. The two mRNA-COVID-19 vaccines approved by the FDA in 2021, the Pfizer-BioNTech COVID-19 Vaccine and the Moderna COVID-19 vaccine, are made up of a single mRNA encoding for the full-length SARS-CoV-2 spike glycoprotein (S) encapsulated in lipid nanoparticles (LNPs) that protect RNA from degradation by RNAses and enable transfection of host cells after intramuscular delivery. The lipid components of the nanocarrier are ALC-0315 (4-hydroxybutyl) azanediyl)bis(hexane-6,1-diyl)bis(2-hexyldecanoate), ALC-0159 (2-[(poly-ethylene glycol)-2000]-N,N-di-tetradecyl acetamide), 1,2-distearoyl-sn-glycero-3-phosphocholine (DSPC), cholesterol for the Pfizer-BioNTech COVID-19 vaccine, and PEG 2000, dimyristoyl glycerol, DSPC, cholesterol and SM-102 for the Moderna COVID-19 vaccine.

As mentioned in Section 4, cationic cSLNs were developed to correct important drawbacks that other nanostructured systems, such as emulsions, liposomes, and polymeric nanoparticles, present in the delivery of genes and/or drugs (i.e., less transfection efficiency, less stability, scale-up difficulties, high costs) [195-197].

Therefore, cSLNs are considered one of the most promising non-viral vectors for nucleic acid delivery and have been widely studied and applied for the delivery of siRNA, mRNA, and pDNA [198-200]. cSLNs offer unique properties that make them especially attractive compared to other types of nanocarrier systems; such as their small size and large surface area, the use of biocompatible excipients that minimize the risk of toxicity, the possibility of being administered by multiple routes (intramuscular, intravenous, nasal, ocular, oral, pulmonary, topical), their capacity to transfect DNA and RNA *in vitro* and *in vivo* with high efficiency, their safe and robust manufacturing process allowing efficient scaling for production at the industrial level, capacity for sterilization by various and non-destructive methods, freeze-drying and storage stability [201]. SLNs have also received increasing attention in recent years as a delivery system for peptides, proteins, antigens, among other bioactive molecules [202].

However, the main drawback of cSLN systems is their tendency to polydispersion and aggregation during short and medium-term storage [203]. Recently, Suñé-Pou et al. proposed the incorporation of cholesteryl oleate (CO), a derivative of cholesterol, into the formulation of cSLNs to improve cytotoxicity and transfection efficiency as a novel strategy for the development of highly efficient and biocompatible therapeutic transporters [204]. Likewise, to improve the ability of cSLNs to transfect cells, the incorporation of the protamine (P) polypeptide has also been proposed [205].

As a strategy to be used as nucleic acid-based vaccines, various modifications are still being investigated and made in the formulation of different cSLNs to improve their transfection efficiency and, therefore, the strength of the immune response triggered. For instance, Francis et al. designed an adjuvant cSLN platform containing monophosphoryl lipid A (MPLA), a TLR4 agonist, to deliver DNA encoding a *Helicobacter pylori* antigen. The resulting lipoplexes were biocompatible and stimulated the expression of the pro-inflammatory cytokine tumor necrosis factor-alpha (TNF-α) in a macrophage cell line [206].

Almeida et al., 1997, showed that SLNs constitute a potential carrier system for the delivery of protein-based vaccines, due to the capacity of SLNs to incorporate hydrophobic or hydrophilic proteins fulfilling the requirements for an optimum particulate carrier system. Proteins and antigens intended for both therapeutic and/or prophylactic purposes may be incorporated or adsorbed onto SLNs, and further administered by parenteral routes or by alternative routes such as oral, nasal and pulmonary. The formulation in SLNs confers improved protein stability, avoids proteolytic degradation, as well as sustained release of the incorporated molecules [207]. In this sense, Mishra et al. explored the potential of mannosylated-SLNs as efficient vaccine delivery carrier systems to enhance the loading efficiency of HBsAg and its cellular uptake for developing an improvised vaccine formulation for chronic hepatitis B infection using the subcutaneous route of administration. The *in vitro* T cell proliferation, induction of TH1 type of immune response and more sustained antibody titer suggested the best immunological potential of the system [208]. In addition, an oral formulation of the HBV vaccine using cSLNs that target the M-cells at the mucosa layer was developed by deriving the cSLNs with lipopolysaccharide, producing a required immune effect against the antigen, and even the pathogen [209]. The potential of cSLNs as efficient adjuvants was described for the inactivated foot and mouth disease virus (iFMDV) vaccine aiming at achieving an enhanced cell immune response and humoral immune response, as well as stability of the unstable iFMDV antigen [202].

With regard to mRNA-based vaccines, their ability to elicit both humoral and cellular immunity has led this vaccine platform to emerge as a transformative approach. As mentioned above, and in contrast to plasmid DNA vaccines, mRNA does not need to be transported across the nuclear membrane and can directly induce antigen expression in the cytosol, so that any potential genomic integration is avoided. Moreover, mRNA vaccines induce transient antigen expression, while DNA vaccines provide a long-lasting expression, thus mimicking an acute viral infection. Although a transitory gene expression might be desirable as it minimizes potential risks of genetic transformation, this inevitably affects mRNA potency, thus necessitating a dose increase [210]. One strategy to augment mRNA performance is to include genetic elements that enable self-amplification (i.e., self-amplifying mRNA (SAM)), hence allowing SAM vaccines to self-amplify over time and consequently inducing more potent immune responses compared to conventional non-amplifying mRNA vaccines [211].

Table 11. Different SLN formulations used for protein and genetic vaccines

Biological	Excipient formulation	Method of preparation	Particle size (nm ± SD)	Adsorption/ Entrapment efficiency (wt %± SD)	Advantages	References
Hepatitis B surface antigen (HBsAg)	Tristearin, Tween™ 80, Monomannosyl-dioleoyl glycerol conjugate	Solvent injection	96.6 ± 2.1	64.53 ± 2.21	Compared to soluble HBsAg; SLNs, particularly the mannosylated formulation, showed better cellular uptake, lesser cytotoxicity and induction of a greater TH1 type of immune response. They also showed better immunological potential by producing sustained antibody titer.	Mishra et al. [208]
	Tristearin, stearylamine, lactose monohydrate, sodium alginate, lipopolysaccharide, Tween™ 80	Solvent injection	313. 82 ± 2.68	n.a.	Effective delivery of antigen through the mucosal oral route. Large amount of antigen can be delivered through SLNs. The association of SLNs to the mucosal M-cells of mice showed better release in comparison to HBsAg alone. Another advantage of the developed nanoformulation was the protection of vaccines against gastric acid along with M-cell targeting.	Saraf et al. [209]

Table 11. (Continued)

Biological	Excipient formulation	Method of preparation	Particle size (nm ± SD)	Adsorption/ Entrapment efficiency (wt %± SD)	Advantages	References
Inactivated foot and mouth disease virus (iFMDV)	Compritol 888 ATO, N-[1-(2,3-Dioleoyloxy) propyl]-N,N,N trimethylammonium chloride, dimethyl dioctadecylammonium bromide, cetyl trimethyl ammonium bromide	O/W emulsion	208.9 ± 2.7 to 254.0 ± 2.6	16.0 to 87.8	cSLNs promoted the uptake of iFMDV by bone-marrow-derived dendritic cells and their activation. cSLN significantly enhanced the proliferation and differentiation of central and effector memory T cells and displayed humoral immunity compared to the adjuvant ISA 206 with improved specific serum antibody levels. Hence, cSLNs might be a promising adjuvant to be applied to iFMDV vaccine.	Li et al. [202]
Self-amplifying mRNA (SAM) encoding rabies virus glycoprotein G	Tristearin, 1,2-dioleoyl-3-trimethylammonium-propane (DOTAP) or dimethyldioctadecylammonium bromide, 1,2-dimyristoyl-rac-glycero-3-methoxypolyethylene glycol-2000	Microfluidic mixer and microfluidization	120 ± 2 to 187 ± 17	99 ± 0.1	Delivery system of SAM. *In vivo*, DOTAP NPs are effective in inducing robust immune responses in mice, with comparable potency to the commercial vaccine Rabipur and the benchmark CNE56.	Anderluzzi et al. [213]

Biological	Excipient formulation	Method of preparation	Particle size (nm ± SD)	Adsorption/ Entrapment efficiency (wt %± SD)	Advantages	References
DNA encoding the Urease A (UreA) antigen from *Helicobacter pylori*	Cholesteryl oleate, glyceryl trioleate,1,2-Dioleoyl-sn-glycero-3-phosphoethanolamine, 3-sn-phosphatidyl-ethanolamine, cholesterol, 3ß-[N-(N',N'-dimethylaminoethane)-carbamoyl]cholesterol hydrochloride, lipid monophosphoryl lipid A from Salmonella enterica serotype Minnesota Re 595 (adjuvant)	Solvent-emulsification	74.67 ± 39.93	n.a.	Cellular uptake studies confirmed particle uptake within 3 h, and intracellular localization within endosomal compartments. *In vitro* studies confirmed the ability of SLNs to stimulate the expression of pro-inflammatory cytokine TNF-α in human macrophage-like Tohoku Hospital Pediatrics-1 (THP-1) cells. Lipoplexes were found to be biocompatible and could be efficiently transfected into murine immune cells for the expression of recombinant *H. pylori* antigen Urease A, demonstrating their potential as a DNA vaccine delivery system.	Francis et al. [206]
DNA expressing a human multiple epitope gag protein (pHIS-HIV-hugag)	Cetylpalmitate, Tween™ 80, Span™ 85, dimethyldioctadecyl ammonium bromide (DDAB), cholesterol	Hot high-pressure homogenization	135 ± 1 to 191 ± 2	n.a.	The SLN cytotoxicity test showed that HeLa cells could tolerate SLNs in a range of 100 to 200 mg/ml.	Asasutjarit et al. [201]

Table 11. (Continued)

Biological	Excipient formulation	Method of preparation	Particle size (nm ± SD)	Adsorption/ Entrapment efficiency (wt %± SD)	Advantages	References
					The results of the transfection study of SLNs at a concentration of 200 mg/ml showed the potential use of SLNs as *in vitro* pHIS-HIV-hugag transfection vectors.	
DNA encoding cysteine proteinases type I, II and III of *Leishmania major*	Cetyl palmitate, Tween™ 80, cholesterol, N-[1-(2,3-Dioleoyloxy) propyl]-N,N,N trimethylammonium chloride (DOTAP), sodium dodecyl sulfate	Hot high-shear homogenization	240± 12 to 250± 15	n.a.	In a murine model of *L. major* infection, SLNs showed a promising role as an adjuvant to enhance a stronger immune response against this infection. The mean average of parasite load reduction for DNA vaccination regimens was determined to be 59.24%. In this study, the percentage of parasite inhibition by DNA vaccination technology could be increased up to 86.3%.	Doroud et al. [214]
DNA encoding proteins A3 and cysteine proteases types I and II of Leishmania infantum	N-[1-(2,3-Dioleoyloxy) propyl]-N,N,N trimethylammonium chloride (DOTAP)	O/W emulsion	241±12	n.a.	The vaccine formulation generates protective immunity with high levels of IFN-γ and lower levels of IL-10 production, leading to a strong Th1 immune response. This DNA vaccine can be protective against visceral leishmaniasis in mice.	Saljoughian et al.[215]

Table 12. Current clinical trials of LPN–mRNA vaccines against some infectious diseases

Company	Name	Disease	Encoded proteins	ClinicalTrials.gov Identifier	Phase
Pfizer/BioNTech	BNT162b2	COVID-19	The viral spike glycoprotein (S)	NCT04588480	Phase II
Moderna/ BARDA/NIAID	mRNA-1273	COVID-19	The prefusion stabilized spike glycoprotein (S)	NCT04470427	Phase III
CureVac AG	mRNA CV7202	Rabies	Rabies virus glycoprotein G (RABV-G)	NCT03713086	Phase I
Moderna/ BARDA	mRNA-1893	Zika	Zika virus pre-membrane and envelope glycoproteins with a JEV leader sequence	NCT04064905	Phase I
Moderna/BARDA	mRNA-1325	Zika	Zika virus antigen pre-membrane and envelope glycoproteins	NCT03014089	Phase I
Moderna	mRNA-1647 and mRNA-1443	Cytomegalovirus(CMV) disease	mRNA-1647: gB (1 mRNA), pentameric complex (5 mRNAs), and mRNA-1443 encoding the pp65 T cell antigen of CMV	NCT03382405	Phase I
Moderna	mRNA-1653	Human metapneumovirus and human parainfluenza virus type 3 (hMPV and PIV3, respectively) diseases	MPV and PIV3 F glycoproteins	NCT03392389	Phase I
Moderna (Valneva)	mRNA-1440	Influenza H10N8	Hemagglutinin	NCT03076385	Phase I
Moderna	mRNA-1851	Influenza H7N9	Hemagglutinin	NCT03345043	Phase I

As with other nucleic acid-based technologies, SAM is prone to enzymatic degradation once injected into the body. In addition, the intrinsic hydrophilic nature and high molecular weight of SAM, challenges its capacity to cross the cell membrane and traverse the endosome for effective delivery to the cytoplasm. Several studies have reported enhanced immunogenicity when SAM vaccines are delivered by a particulate delivery system [212]. Of the systems tested, LNPs are the most advanced in enabling the clinical potential of genetic drugs, such as siRNA and mRNA, with several siRNA-LNP systems already in clinical trials as antiviral, anticancer and genetic disorder therapies. Anderluzzi et al. have investigated SLNs as non-viral vectors for the delivery of SAM encoding rabies virus glycoprotein G. Their immunogenicity was compared to that of the licensed rabies vaccine Rabipur and the cationic nanoemulsion (CNE56) as benchmarks for the rabies vaccine and mRNA delivery, respectively. *In vivo*, SLNs showed to be effective in inducing robust immune responses in mice, with comparable potency to the commercial vaccine Rabipur and CNE56 [213]. DNA-based vaccines using SLNs were also developed against *Helicobacter pylori* infection and cutaneous/visceral leishmaniasis [214, 215].

Table 11 shows some examples of the vaccines developed using SLNs. Table 12 lists those vaccines that are currently under evaluation in clinical trials against some infectious diseases (https://clinicaltrials.gov/, accessed in October 2022).

Conclusion

Infectious diseases remain the major causes of morbidity and mortality.

One of the steps that should be taken for reducing the morbidity and mortality risk related to infectious diseases, includes their prevention, treatment and control.

Few drugs are available for the management of NTDs, and some of these neglected entities do not even have a specific drug treatment yet, as is the case of dengue and chikungunya. Despite the fact that few of the available drugs are considered effective, their efficacy depends on multiple factors, such as the presence of MDR, microorganism species, and host immune status. Moreover, the high incidence of side effects associated with toxicity using many of these drugs, such as pentavalent antimonial drugs or AmB for leishmaniasis contributes to limit their use in clinical practice. The lack of safe, effective and affordable medicines is a key contributing factor to improve the situation and control NTDs.

Considering that drug discovery involves a very long and expensive process, and that pharmaceutical companies are not ensured sufficient economic profits from drugs to mitigate NTDs, little motivation exists to encourage their commercial interest for research and development.

An alternative way could be based on the development of technologies to improve drug delivery for treating numerous infectious diseases, including those considered NTDs.

Nanotechnology has emerged as the novel magic bullet of the 21st century for the treatment of several human illnesses, including infectious diseases.

Since the approval of the first antimicrobial nanomedicine, AmBisome™ 25 years ago, significant efforts have been made towards the development of novel drug formulations against different infectious diseases, including some NTDs using lipid- or polymer-based nanocarriers. Among them, several nanoformulations against deep mycoses, TB, helminthiasis, malaria and leishmaniasis have been developed.

To date, only 11 nanomedicines (ADCs) against infectious diseases have been approved and reached clinical practice, whereas many other nanoformulated versions of existing drugs are under development or evaluation in ongoing clinical trials. This poor clinical translation is associated to failures in transferring true clinical benefits to patients. For instance, several nanopharmaceuticals were unable to demonstrate significant improvements in terms of efficacy compared to standard therapies; in other cases, the toxicity profile of a drug was improved with another drug or nanoformulation.

As an emerging new field, nanomedicine and its further therapeutic application in different infectious diseases is blooming, with successful contributions such as AmBisome™ and Arikayce™ and some stumbling blocks in the way, as was the disappointing clinical outcome of Pulmaquin™, a liposome formulation of ciprofloxacine that was not granted approval by the FDA.

Among several nanoparticulate drug delivery systems, SLNs constitute a promising platform for the encapsulation of lipophilic and hydrophilic drugs to achieve improved solubility (in the case of poorly water-soluble drugs), target accumulation to specific cells, tissues or organs, reduced toxicity and overcome MDR. Hence, SLNs have all the potential to become an innovative class of therapeutics or vaccine delivery systems for numerous infectious diseases, although liposomes, nanocrystals and polymeric formulations are currently the nanoformulations that have advanced the most in clinical development.

To achieve this goal, fundamental research should continue to explore new nanomaterials and possibilities to improve the therapeutic efficacy and applicability of both SLNs and approved drugs.

Finally, designing and implementing nanotechnologies at reasonable costs and making them affordable to people in developing countries are key ethical and scientific issues involved in guaranteeing and humanizing the right to health.

References

[1] WHO, *The top 10 causes of death.* https://www.who.int/news-room/fact-sheets/detail/the-top-10-causes-of-death (accessed 4 October 2022).

[2] Basak S, Singh P, Rajurkar M. Multidrug Resistant and Extensively Drug Resistant Bacteria: A Study. *J Pathog.* 2016; 2016:4065603. doi: 10.1155/2016/4065603.

[3] WHO, *Antimicrobial resistance: global report on surveillance 2014.* https://www.who.int/antimicrobial-resistance/publications/surveillancereport/en/ (accessed 9 September 2022).

[4] The Interagency Coordination Group on Antimicrobial Resistance (IACG). 2019. No time to wait: Securing the future from drug-resistant infections. Report to the Secretary-General of the United Nations. https://www.who.int/docs/default-source/documents/no-time-to-waitsecuring-the-future-from-drug-resistant-infe ctions-en.pdf?sfvrsn=5b424d7_6 (accessed 13 August 2021).

[5] Arias CA, Murray BE. Antibiotic-resistant bugs in the 21st century--a clinical super-challenge. *N Engl J Med.* 2009;360(5):439-43. doi: 10.1056/NEJMp08046 51.

[6] Sharma A. Antimicrobial resistance: no action today, no cure tomorrow. *Indian J Med Microbiol.* 2011;29(2):91-2. doi: 10.4103/0255-0857.81774.

[7] Kostakioti M, Hadjifrangiskou M, Hultgren SJ. Bacterial biofilms: development, dispersal, and therapeutic strategies in the dawn of the postantibiotic era. *Cold Spring Harb Perspect Med.* 2013;3(4):a010306. doi: 10.1101/cshperspect.a0103 06.

[8] Veerachamy S, Yarlagadda T, Manivasagam G, Yarlagadda PK. Bacterial adherence and biofilm formation on medical implants: a review. *Proc Inst Mech Eng H.* 2014;228(10):1083-99. doi: 10.1177/0954411914556137.

[9] Bjarnsholt T. The role of bacterial biofilms in chronic infections. *APMIS Suppl.* 2013;136:1-51. doi: 10.1111/apm.12099.

[10] Jamal M, Ahmad W, Andleeb S, Jalil F, Imran M, Nawaz MA, Hussain T, Ali M, Rafiq M, Kamil MA. Bacterial biofilm and associated infections. *J Chin Med Assoc.* 2018;81(1):7-11. doi: 10.1016/j.jcma.2017.07.012.

[11] Davies D. Understanding biofilm resistance to antibacterial agents. *Nat Rev Drug Discov.* 2003;2(2):114-22. doi: 10.1038/nrd1008.

[12] Høiby N, Bjarnsholt T, Givskov M, Molin S, Ciofu O. Antibiotic resistance of bacterial biofilms. *Int J Antimicrob Agents.* 2010;35(4):322-32. doi: 10.1016/j.ijantimicag.2009.12.011.

[13] Chiappetta DA, Sosnik A. Poly(ethylene oxide)-poly(propylene oxide) block copolymer micelles as drug delivery agents: improved hydrosolubility, stability and bioavailability of drugs. *Eur J Pharm Biopharm.* 2007;66(3):303-17. doi: 10.1016/j.ejpb.2007.03.022.

[14] Limeres MJ, Moretton MA, Bernabeu E, Chiappetta DA, Cuestas ML. Thinking small, doing big: Current success and future trends in drug delivery systems for improving cancer therapy with special focus on liver cancer. *Mater Sci Eng C Mater Biol Appl.* 2019;95:328-341. doi: 10.1016/j.msec.2018.11.001.

[15] Chiappetta DA, Degrossi J, Teves S, D'Aquino M, Bregni C, Sosnik A. Triclosan-loaded poloxamine micelles for enhanced topical antibacterial activity against biofilm. *Eur J Pharm Biopharm.* 2008;69(2):535-45. doi: 10.1016/j.ejpb.2007.11.021.

[16] Seremeta KP, Chiappetta DA, Sosnik A. Poly(ε-caprolactone), Eudragit® RS 100 and poly(ε-caprolactone)/Eudragit® RS 100 blend submicron particles for the sustained release of the antiretroviral efavirenz. *Colloids Surf B Biointerfaces.* 2013;102:441-9. doi: 10.1016/j.colsurfb.2012.06.038.

[17] Moretton MA, Chiappetta DA, Andrade F, das Neves J, Ferreira D, Sarmento B, Sosnik A. Hydrolyzed galactomannan-modified nanoparticles and flower-like polymeric micelles for the active targeting of rifampicin to macrophages. *J Biomed Nanotechnol.* 2013;9(6):1076-87. doi: 10.1166/jbn.2013.1600.

[18] Salerno C, Chiappetta DA, Arechavala A, Gorzalczany S, Scioscia SL, Bregni C. Lipid-based microtubes for topical delivery of amphotericin B. *Colloids Surf B Biointerfaces.* 2013;107:160-6. doi: 10.1016/j.colsurfb.2013.02.001.

[19] Chiappetta DA, Hocht C, Opezzo JA, Sosnik A. Intranasal administration of antiretroviral-loaded micelles for anatomical targeting to the brain in HIV. *Nanomedicine* (Lond). 2013 Feb;8(2):223-37. doi: 10.2217/nnm.12.104.

[20] Moretton MA, Taira C, Flor S, Bernabeu E, Lucangioli S, Höcht C, Chiappetta DA. Novel nelfinavir mesylate loaded d-α-tocopheryl polyethylene glycol 1000 succinate micelles for enhanced pediatric anti-HIV therapy: In vitro characterization and in vivo evaluation. *Colloids Surf B Biointerfaces.* 2014;123:302-10. doi: 10.1016/j.colsurfb.2014.09.031.

[21] Moretton MA, Cohen L, Lepera L, Bernabeu E, Taira C, Höcht C, Chiappetta DA. Enhanced oral bioavailability of nevirapine within micellar nanocarriers compared with Viramune(®). *Colloids Surf B Biointerfaces.* 2014;122:56-65. doi: 10.1016/j.colsurfb.2014.06.046.

[22] Tshweu L, Katata L, Kalombo L, Chiappetta DA, Hocht C, Sosnik A, Swai H. Enhanced oral bioavailability of the antiretroviral efavirenz encapsulated in poly(epsilon-caprolactone) nanoparticles by a spray-drying method. *Nanomedicine* (Lond). 2014;9(12):1821-33. doi: 10.2217/nnm.13.167.

[23] Moretton MA, Cagel M, Bernabeu E, Gonzalez L, Chiappetta DA. Nanopolymersomes as potential carriers for rifampicin pulmonary delivery. *Colloids Surf B Biointerfaces.* 2015;136:1017-25. doi: 10.1016/j.colsurfb.2015.10.049.

[24] Kheirollahpour M, Mehrabi M, Dounighi NM, Mohammadi M, Masoudi A. Nanoparticles and Vaccine Development. *Pharm Nanotechnol.* 2020;8(1):6-21. doi: 10.2174/2211738507666191024162042.

[25] Cuestas ML, Castillo AI, Sosnik A, Mathet VL. Downregulation of mdr1 and abcg2 genes is a mechanism of inhibition of efflux pumps mediated by polymeric amphiphiles. *Bioorg Med Chem Lett.* 2012;22(21):6577-9. doi: 10.1016/j.bmcl.2012.09.012.

[26] Zhou Y, Zhang K, Yin X, Nie Q, Ma Y. HIV-1 Tat Protein Enhances Expression and Function of Breast Cancer Resistance Protein. *AIDS Res Hum Retroviruses.* 2016;32(1):1-3. doi: 10.1089/aid.2015.0117.

[27] Roma MI, Hocht C, Chiappetta DA, Di Gennaro SS, Minoia JM, Bramuglia GF, Rubio MC, Sosnik A, Peroni RN. Tetronic® 904-containing polymeric micelles overcome the overexpression of ABCG2 in the blood-brain barrier of rats and boost the penetration of the antiretroviral efavirenz into the CNS. *Nanomedicine* (Lond). 2015;10(15):2325-37. doi: 10.2217/NNM.15.77.

[28] Pelgrift RY, Friedman AJ. Nanotechnology as a therapeutic tool to combat microbial resistance. *Adv Drug Deliv Rev.* 2013;65(13-14):1803-15. doi: 10.1016/j.addr.2013.07.011.

[29] Baek JS, Cho CW. Surface modification of solid lipid nanoparticles for oral delivery of curcumin: Improvement of bioavailability through enhanced cellular uptake, and lymphatic uptake. *Eur J Pharm Biopharm.* 2017;117:132-140. doi: 10.1016/j.ejpb.2017.04.013.

[30] Martins S, Costa-Lima S, Carneiro T, Cordeiro-da-Silva A, Souto EB, Ferreira DC. Solid lipid nanoparticles as intracellular drug transporters: an investigation of the uptake mechanism and pathway. *Int J Pharm.* 2012;430(1-2):216-27. doi: 10.1016/j.ijpharm.2012.03.032.

[31] Rostami E, Kashanian S, Azandaryani AH, Faramarzi H, Dolatabadi JE, Omidfar K. Drug targeting using solid lipid nanoparticles. *Chem Phys Lipids.* 2014;181:56-61. doi: 10.1016/j.chemphyslip.2014.03.006.

[32] Karamanou M, Panayiotakopoulos G, Tsoucalas G, Kousoulis AA, Androutsos G. From miasmas to germs: a historical approach to theories of infectious disease transmission. *Infez Med.* 2012;20(1):58-62.

[33] WHO. *Coronavirus disease (COVID-19) pandemic.* https://www.who.int/emergencies/diseases/novel-coronavirus-2019 (accessed 4 October 2022).

[34] Lane N. The unseen world: reflections on Leeuwenhoek (1677) 'Concerning little animals'. *Philos Trans R Soc Lond B Biol Sci.* 2015;370(1666):20140344. doi: 10.1098/rstb.2014.0344.

[35] Maloy S, Schaechter M. The era of microbiology: a golden phoenix. *Int Microbiol.* 2006;9(1):1-7.

[36] Standing up to infectious disease. *Nat Microbiol.* 4(1) (2019). https://doi.org/10.1038/s41564-018-0331-3.

[37] Hay SI, Battle KE, Pigott DM, Smith DL, Moyes CL, Bhatt S, Brownstein JS, Collier N, Myers MF, George DB, Gething PW. Global mapping of infectious disease. *Philos Trans R Soc Lond B Biol Sci.* 2013;368(1614):20120250. doi: 10.1098/rstb.2012.0250.

[38] WHO, *Control of Neglected Tropical Diseases.* https://www.who.int/neglected_diseases/diseases/en/ (accessed 9 December 2019).

[39] Molyneux D. Neglected tropical diseases. *Community Eye Health.* 2013;26(82):21-4.

[40] Cuestas ML. Therapy of Chronic Hepatitis C in the Era of Nanotechnology: Drug Delivery Systems and Liver Targeting. *Mini Rev Med Chem.* 2017;17(3):295-304. doi: 10.2174/1389557516666161019152716.

[41] Feynman R.P. There's plenty of room at the bottom. *Eng and Sci* 23(5) (1960). 22-36.

[42] Bernabeu E, Cagel M, Lagomarsino E, Moretton M, Chiappetta DA. Paclitaxel: What has been done and the challenges remain ahead. *Int J Pharm.* 2017;526(1-2):474-495. doi: 10.1016/j.ijpharm.2017.05.016.

[43] Schütz CA, Juillerat-Jeanneret L, Mueller H, Lynch I, Riediker M; NanoImpactNet Consortium. Therapeutic nanoparticles in clinics and under clinical evaluation. *Nanomedicine* (Lond). 2013;8(3):449-67. doi: 10.2217/nnm.13.8.

[44] Ge Y, Li S, Wang S, Moore R. *Nanomedicine.* Principles and Perspectives, Springer, Otawa, 2014.

[45] Strebhardt K, Ullrich A. Paul Ehrlich's magic bullet concept: 100 years of progress. *Nat Rev Cancer.* 2008;8(6):473-80. doi: 10.1038/nrc2394.

[46] Cagel M, Grotz E, Bernabeu E, Moretton MA, Chiappetta DA. Doxorubicin: nanotechnological overviews from bench to bedside. *Drug Discov Today.* 2017;22(2):270-281. doi: 10.1016/j.drudis.2016.11.005.

[47] Andrade F, Rafael D, Videira M, Ferreira D, Sosnik A, Sarmento B. Nanotechnology and pulmonary delivery to overcome resistance in infectious diseases. *Adv Drug Deliv Rev.* 2013;65(13-14):1816-27. doi: 10.1016/j.addr.2013.07.020.

[48] Ruge CA, Schaefer UF, Herrmann J, Kirch J, Cañadas O, Echaide M, Pérez-Gil J, Casals C, Müller R, Lehr CM. The interplay of lung surfactant proteins and lipids assimilates the macrophage clearance of nanoparticles. *PLoS One.* 2012; 7(7):e40775. doi: 10.1371/journal.pone.0040775.

[49] Velasco-Aguirre C, Morales-Zavala F, Salas-Huenuleo E, Gallardo-Toledo E, Andonie O, Muñoz L, Rojas X, Acosta G, Sánchez-Navarro M, Giralt E, Araya E, Albericio F, Kogan MJ. Improving gold nanorod delivery to the central nervous system by conjugation to the shuttle Angiopep-2. *Nanomedicine* (Lond). 2017;12(20):2503-2517. doi: 10.2217/nnm-2017-0181.

[50] Ahsan F, Rivas IP, Khan MA, Torres Suarez AI. Targeting to macrophages: role of physicochemical properties of particulate carriers--liposomes and microspheres--on the phagocytosis by macrophages. *J Control Release.* 2002;79(1-3):29-40. doi: 10.1016/s0168-3659(01)00549-1.

[51] Halwani AA. Development of Pharmaceutical Nanomedicines: From the Bench to the Market. *Pharmaceutics.* 2022;14(1):106. doi: 10.3390/pharmaceutics14010106.

[52] Tapeinos C, Battaglini M, Ciofani G. Advances in the design of solid lipid nanoparticles and nanostructured lipid carriers for targeting brain diseases. *J Control Release.* 2017;264:306-332. doi: 10.1016/j.jconrel.2017.08.033.

[53] Mishra V, Bansal KK, Verma A, Yadav N, Thakur S, Sudhakar K, Rosenholm JM. Solid Lipid Nanoparticles: Emerging Colloidal Nano Drug Delivery Systems. *Pharmaceutics.* 2018;10(4):191. doi: 10.3390/pharmaceutics10040191.

[54] Mukherjee S, Ray S, Thakur RS. Solid lipid nanoparticles: a modern formulation approach in drug delivery system. *Indian J Pharm Sci.* 2009;71(4):349-58. doi: 10.4103/0250-474X.57282.

[55] Naseri N, Valizadeh H, Zakeri-Milani P. Solid Lipid Nanoparticles and Nanostructured Lipid Carriers: Structure, Preparation and Application. *Adv Pharm Bull.* 2015;5(3):305-13. doi: 10.15171/apb.2015.043.

[56] Müller RH, Radtke M, Wissing SA. Nanostructured lipid matrices for improved microencapsulation of drugs. *Int J Pharm.* 2002;242(1-2):121-8. doi: 10.1016/s0378-5173(02)00180-1.

[57] Das S, Ng WK, Tan RB. Are nanostructured lipid carriers (NLCs) better than solid lipid nanoparticles (SLNs): development, characterizations and comparative evaluations of clotrimazole-loaded SLNs and NLCs? *Eur J Pharm Sci.* 2012;47(1):139-51. doi: 10.1016/j.ejps.2012.05.010.

[58] Li F, Wang Y, Liu Z, Lin X, He H, Tang X. Formulation and characterization of bufadienolides-loaded nanostructured lipid carriers. *Drug Dev Ind Pharm.* 2010;36(5):508-17. doi: 10.3109/03639040903264397.

[59] CDC, *Fungal Diseases.* https://www.cdc.gov/fungal/about-fungal-diseases.html (accessed 16 December 2019).

[60] Brown GD, Denning DW, Gow NA, Levitz SM, Netea MG, White TC. Hidden killers: human fungal infections. *Sci Transl Med.* 2012;4(165):165rv13. doi: 10.1126/scitranslmed.3004404.

[61] Ramana KV, Kandi S, Bharatkumar P, Sharada CHV, Rao R, Mani R, Rao SD. Invasive fungal infections: a comprehensive review. *Am J Infect Dis Microbiol* 1 (2013) 64-69. https://doi.org/10.12691/ajidm-1-4-2.

[62] Goughenour KD, Rappleye CA. Antifungal therapeutics for dimorphic fungal pathogens. *Virulence.* 2017;8(2):211-221. doi: 10.1080/21505594.2016.1235653.

[63] Souza AC, Amaral AC. Antifungal Therapy for Systemic Mycosis and the Nanobiotechnology Era: Improving Efficacy, Biodistribution and Toxicity. *Front Microbiol.* 2017;8:336. doi: 10.3389/fmicb.2017.00336.

[64] Pappas PG. Antifungal clinical trials and guidelines: what we know and do not know. *Cold Spring Harb Perspect Med.* 2014;4(11):a019745. doi: 10.1101/cshperspect.a019745.

[65] Proffitt RT, Satorius A, Chiang SM, Sullivan L, Adler-Moore JP. Pharmacology and toxicology of a liposomal formulation of amphotericin B (AmBisome) in rodents. *J Antimicrob Chemother.* 1991;28 Suppl B:49-61. doi: 10.1093/jac/28.suppl_b.49.

[66] Clark JM, Whitney RR, Olsen SJ, George RJ, Swerdel MR, Kunselman L, Bonner DP. Amphotericin B lipid complex therapy of experimental fungal infections in mice. *Antimicrob Agents Chemother.* 1991;35(4):615-21. doi: 10.1128/AAC.35.4.615.

[67] Guo LSS, Fielding RM, Lasic DD, Hamilton RL, Mufson D. Novel antifungal drug delivery: stable amphotericin B-cholesteryl sulfate discs. *Int J Pharm.* 1991; 75:45–54. doi: 10.1016/0378-5173(91)90249-N.

[68] Nett JE, Andes DR. Antifungal agents: Spectrum of activity, pharmacology, and clinical indications. *Infect Dis Clin North Am.* 2016; 30(1):51–83. doi: 10.1016/j.idc.2015.10.012.

[69] Hargrove TY, Garvey EP, Hoekstra WJ, Yates CM, Wawrzak Z, Rachakonda G, Villalta F, Lepesheva GI. Crystal structure of the new investigational drug candidate VT-1598 in complex with *Aspergillus fumigatus* sterol 14α-demethylase provides insights into its broad-spectrum antifungal activity. *Antimicrob Agents Chemother.* 2017;61(7):e00570-17. doi: 10.1128/AAC.00570-17.

[70] Peyton LR, Gallagher S, Hashemzadeh M. Triazole antifungals: a review. *Drugs Today (Barc).* 2015;51(12):705-18. doi: 10.1358/dot.2015.51.12.2421058.

[71] Sucher AJ, Chahine EB, Balcer HE. Echinocandins: the newest class of antifungals. *Ann Pharmacother.* 2009;43(10):1647-57. doi: 10.1345/aph.1M237.

[72] Polvi EJ, Li X, O'Meara TR, Leach MD, Cowen LE. Opportunistic yeast pathogens: reservoirs, virulence mechanisms, and therapeutic strategies. *Cell Mol Life Sci.* 2015;72(12):2261-87. doi: 10.1007/s00018-015-1860-z.

[73] Resendiz Sharpe A, Lagrou K, Meis JF, Chowdhary A, Lockhart SR, Verweij PE; ISHAM/ECMM *Aspergillus* Resistance Surveillance working group. Triazole resistance surveillance in *Aspergillus fumigatus. Med Mycol.* 2018;56(suppl_1):83-92. doi: 10.1093/mmy/myx144.

[74] Bianco, MA, Gallarate, M, Trotta, M, & Battaglia, L. Amphotericin B loaded SLN prepared with the coacervation technique. *J. Drug Del. Sci. Tech.* 2010; 20(3): 187–91.

[75] Patel PA, Patravale VB. AmbiOnp: solid lipid nanoparticles of amphotericin B for oral administration. *J Biomed Nanotechnol.* 2011;7(5):632-9. doi: 10.1166/jbn.2011.1332.

[76] Chaudhari MB, Desai PP, Patel PA, Patravale VB. Solid lipid nanoparticles of amphotericin B (AmbiOnp): *in vitro* and *in vivo* assessment towards safe and effective oral treatment module. *Drug Deliv Transl Res.* 2016;6(4):354-64. doi: 10.1007/s13346-015-0267-6.

[77] Aljaeid BM, Hosny KM. Miconazole-loaded solid lipid nanoparticles: formulation and evaluation of a novel formula with high bioavailability and antifungal activity. *Int J Nanomedicine.* 2016;11:441-7. doi: 10.2147/IJN.S100625.

[78] Araujo VHS, Delello Di Filippo L, Duarte JL, Spósito L, Camargo BAF, da Silva PB, Chorilli M. Exploiting solid lipid nanoparticles and nanostructured lipid carriers for drug delivery against cutaneous fungal infections. *Crit Rev Microbiol.* 2021;47(1):79-90. doi: 10.1080/1040841X.2020.1843399.

[79] Butani D, Yewale C, Misra A. Topical Amphotericin B solid lipid nanoparticles: Design and development. *Colloids Surf B Biointerfaces.* 2016;139:17-24. doi: 10.1016/j.colsurfb.2015.07.032.

[80] Moazeni M, Kelidari HR, Saeedi M, Morteza-Semnani K, Nabili M, Gohar AA, Akbari J, Lotfali E, Nokhodchi A. Time to overcome fluconazole resistant *Candida* isolates: Solid lipid nanoparticles as a novel antifungal drug delivery system. *Colloids Surf B Biointerfaces.* 2016;142:400-407. doi: 10.1016/j.colsurfb.2016.03.013.

[81] Gupta M, Vyas SP. Development, characterization and *in vivo* assessment of effective lipidic nanoparticles for dermal delivery of fluconazole against cutaneous candidiasis. *Chem Phys Lipids.* 2012;165(4):454-61. doi: 10.1016/j.chemphyslip.2012.01.006.

[82] Gupta M, Tiwari S, Vyas SP. Influence of various lipid core on characteristics of SLNs designed for topical delivery of fluconazole against cutaneous candidiasis. *Pharm Dev Technol.* 2013;18(3):550-9. doi: 10.3109/10837450.2011.598161.

[83] El-Housiny S, Shams Eldeen MA, El-Attar YA, Salem HA, Attia D, Bendas ER, El-Nabarawi MA. Fluconazole-loaded solid lipid nanoparticles topical gel for treatment of pityriasis versicolor: formulation and clinical study. *Drug Deliv.* 2018;25(1):78-90. doi: 10.1080/10717544.2017.1413444.

[84] Mirza MA, Panda AK, Asif S, Verma D, Talegaonkar S, Manzoor N, Khan A, Ahmed FJ, Dudeja M, Iqbal Z. A vaginal drug delivery model. *Drug Deliv.* 2016;23(8):3123-3134. doi: 10.3109/10717544.2016.1153749.

[85] Bhalekar MR, Pokharkar V, Madgulkar A, Patil N, Patil N. Preparation and evaluation of miconazole nitrate-loaded solid lipid nanoparticles for topical delivery. *AAPS Pharm Sci Tech.* 2009;10(1):289-96. doi: 10.1208/s12249-009-9199-0.

[86] Jain S, Jain S, Khare P, Gulbake A, Bansal D, Jain SK. Design and development of solid lipid nanoparticles for topical delivery of an anti-fungal agent. *Drug Deliv.* 2010;17(6):443-51. doi: 10.3109/10717544.2010.483252.

[87] Ramasamy, T, Khandasami, US, Ruttala, H, Shanmugam, S. et al. Development of solid lipid nanoparticles enriched hydrogels for topical delivery of anti-fungal agent. *Macromol. Res.* 2012; 20:682–92. doi: 10.1007/s13233-012-0107-1.

[88] Cassano R, Ferrarelli T, Mauro MV, Cavalcanti P, Picci N, Trombino S. Preparation, characterization and in vitro activities evaluation of solid lipid nanoparticles based on PEG-40 stearate for antifungal drugs vaginal delivery. *Drug Deliv.* 2016;23(3):1047-56. doi: 10.3109/10717544.2014.932862.

[89] Souto EB, Müller RH. SLN and NLC for topical delivery of ketoconazole. *J Microencapsul.* 2005;22(5):501-10. doi: 10.1080/02652040500162436.

[90] Souto EB, Wissing SA, Barbosa CM, Müller RH. Development of a controlled release formulation based on SLN and NLC for topical clotrimazole delivery. *Int J Pharm.* 2004;278(1):71-7. doi: 10.1016/j.ijpharm.2004.02.032.

[91] Das S, Ng WK, Tan RB. Sucrose ester stabilized solid lipid nanoparticles and nanostructured lipid carriers. I. Effect of formulation variables on the physicochemical properties, drug release and stability of clotrimazole-loaded

nanoparticles. *Nanotechnology*. 2014;25(10):105101. doi: 10.1088/0957-4484/25/10/105101.

[92] Sanna V, Gavini E, Cossu M, Rassu G, Giunchedi P. Solid lipid nanoparticles (SLN) as carriers for the topical delivery of econazole nitrate: in-vitro characterization, ex-vivo and in-vivo studies. *J Pharm Pharmacol.* 2007;59(8): 1057-64. doi: 10.1211/jpp.59.8.0002.

[93] Aggarwal N, Goindi S. Preparation and in vivo evaluation of solid lipid nanoparticles of griseofulvin for dermal use. *J Biomed Nanotechnol.* 2013;9(4): 564-76. doi: 10.1166/jbn.2013.1569.

[94] Lorwongngam A, Gaysorn C, Dangprasirt P, Kongmuang S. Griseofulvin solid lipid nanoparticles based on microemulsion technique. *Adv Mat Res.* 2011;197-8. doi: 10.4028/www.scientific.net/AMR.197-198.47.

[95] Vaghasiya H, Kumar A, Sawant K. Development of solid lipid nanoparticles based controlled release system for topical delivery of terbinafine hydrochloride. *Eur J Pharm Sci.* 2013 May 13;49(2):311-22. doi: 10.1016/j.ejps.2013.03.013.

[96] Chen YC, Liu DZ, Liu JJ, Chang TW, Ho HO, Sheu MT. Development of terbinafine solid lipid nanoparticles as a topical delivery system. *Int J Nanomedicine.* 2012; 7:4409-18. doi: 10.2147/IJN.S33682.

[97] Mohanty B, Majumdar DK, Mishra SK, Panda AK, Patnaik S. Development and characterization of itraconazole-loaded solid lipid nanoparticles for ocular delivery. *Pharm Dev Technol.* 2015;20(4):458-64. doi: 10.3109/10837450.2014.882935.

[98] Khare A, Singh I, Pawar P, Grover K. Design and evaluation of voriconazole loaded solid lipid nanoparticles for ophthalmic application. *J Drug Deliv.* 2016; 2016:6590361. doi: 10.1155/2016/6590361.

[99] Kumar R, Sinha VR. Solid lipid nanoparticle: an efficient carrier for improved ocular permeation of voriconazole. *Drug Dev Ind Pharm.* 2016;42(12):1956-1967. doi: 10.1080/03639045.2016.1185437.

[100] Pandurangan DK, Bodagala P, Palanirajan VK, Govindaraj S. Formulation and evaluation of voriconazole ophthalmic solid lipid nanoparticles in situ gel. *Int J Pharm Investig.* 2016;6(1):56-62. doi: 10.4103/2230-973X.176488.

[101] Youshia J, Kamel AO, El Shamy A, Mansour S. Design of cationic nanostructured heterolipid matrices for ocular delivery of methazolamide. *Int J Nanomedicine.* 2012;7:2483-96. doi: 10.2147/IJN.S28307.

[102] Mehrabani Yeganeh E, Bagheri H, Mahjub R. Preparation, statistical optimization and *in-vitro* characterization of a dry powder inhaler (DPI) containing solid lipid nanoparticles encapsulating amphotericin B: Ion paired complexes with distearoyl phosphatidylglycerol. *Iran J Pharm Res.* 2020 Summer;19(3):45-62. doi: 10.22037/ijpr.2019.15208.12963.

[103] Oubiña JR. Ébola 2014: drama y esperanza [*Ebola 2014: drama and hope*]. *Rev Argent Microbiol.* 2014;46(4):283-7. doi: 10.1016/S0325-7541(14)70083-5.

[104] Bratanich A. MERS-CoV: transmisión y el papel de nuevas especies hospederas [*MERS-CoV, transmission and the role of new host species*]. *Rev Argent Microbiol.* 2015;47(4):279-81. doi: 10.1016/j.ram.2015.11.001.

[105] Cuestas ML. Desde los astros y el frío hasta el virus pandémico de la influenza A (H1N1): una amenaza permanente para la humanidad [*From stars and cold to the*

pandemic Influenza A (H1N1) virus: A permanent threat to humanity]. *Rev Argent Microbiol.* 2016;48(3):185-186.. doi: 10.1016/j.ram.2016.08.001.

[106] Minassian ML. Virus Zika: Crónica de una pandemia ¿impensada? [*Zika virus: chronicle of an "unexpected" pandemic*]. *Rev Argent Microbiol.* 2016;48(2):97-9. doi: 10.1016/j.ram.2016.06.001.

[107] Cuestas ML, Minassian ML. Virus emergentes y reemergentes: un nuevo reto para la salud mundial del milenio [*Emerging and re-emerging viruses: A new challenge for global health in this millennium*]. *Rev Argent Microbiol.* 2020;52(1):1-3. doi: 10.1016/j.ram.2020.02.001.

[108] Cuestas ML, Rivero CW, Minassian ML, Castillo AI, Gentile EA, Trinks J, León L, Daleoso G, Frider B, Lezama C, Galoppo M, Giacove G, Mathet VL, Oubiña JR. Naturally occurring hepatitis B virus (HBV) variants with primary resistance to antiviral therapy and S-mutants with potential primary resistance to adefovir in Argentina. *Antiviral Res.* 2010;87(1):74-7. doi: 10.1016/j.antiviral.2010.04.005.

[109] De Clercq E, Li G. Approved antiviral drugs over the past 50 years. *Clin Microbiol Rev.* 2016;29(3):695-747. doi: 10.1128/CMR.00102-15.

[110] Parthiban R, Sathishkumar S, Ramakrishnan P. Design and evaluation of acyclovir-loaded solid lipid nanoparticles for sustained release. *Drug Invent* Today. 2020; 14(1), 108-11.

[111] El-Gizawy SA, El-Maghraby GM, Hedaya AA. Formulation of acyclovir-loaded solid lipid nanoparticles: design, optimization, and *in-vitro* characterization. *Pharm Dev Technol.* 2019;24(10):1287-98. doi: 10.1080/10837450.2019.1667385.

[112] Javan F, Vatanara A, Azadmanesh K, Nabi-Meibodi M, Shakouri M. Encapsulation of ritonavir in solid lipid nanoparticles: *in-vitro* anti-HIV-1 activity using lentiviral particles. *J Pharm Pharmacol.* 2017;69(8):1002-1009. doi: 10.1111/jphp.12737.

[113] Alex A, Paul W, Chacko AJ, Sharma CP. Enhanced delivery of lopinavir to the CNS using Compritol-based solid lipid nanoparticles. *Ther Deliv.* 2011;2(1):25-35. doi: 10.4155/tde.10.96.

[114] Chattopadhyay N, Zastre J, Wong HL, Wu XY, Bendayan R. Solid lipid nanoparticles enhance the delivery of the HIV protease inhibitor, atazanavir, by a human brain endothelial cell line. *Pharm Res.* 2008;25(10):2262-71. doi: 10.1007/ s11095-008-9615-2.

[115] Negi JS, Chattopadhyay P, Sharma AK, Ram V. Development and evaluation of glyceryl behenate based solid lipid nanoparticles (SLNs) using hot self-nanoemulsification (SNE) technique. *Arch Pharm Res.* 2014;37(3):361-70. doi: 10. 1007/s12272-013-0154-y.

[116] Gaur PK, Mishra S, Bajpai M, Mishra A. Enhanced oral bioavailability of efavirenz by solid lipid nanoparticles: *in vitro* drug release and pharmacokinetics studies. *Biomed Res Int.* 2014;2014:363404. doi: 10.1155/2014/363404.

[117] Joshy K S, Sharma CP, Kalarikkal N, Sandeep K, Thomas S, Pothen LA. Evaluation of *in-vitro* cytotoxicity and cellular uptake efficiency of zidovudine-loaded solid lipid nanoparticles modified with Aloe Vera in glioma cells. *Mater Sci Eng C Mater Biol Appl.* 2016;66:40-50. doi: 10.1016/j.msec.2016.03.031.

[118] Kuo YC, Wang CC. Cationic solid lipid nanoparticles with cholesterol-mediated surface layer for transporting saquinavir to the brain. *Biotechnol Prog.* 2014; 30(1):198-206. doi: 10.1002/btpr.1834.

[119] Singh S, Dobhal AK, Jain A, Pandit JK, Chakraborty S. Formulation and evaluation of solid lipid nanoparticles of a water soluble drug: Zidovudine. *Chem Pharm Bull* (Tokyo). 2010;58(5):650-5. doi: 10.1248/cpb.58.650.

[120] Sankar V, Nareshkumar PN, Ajitkumar GN, Penmetsa SD, Hariharan S. Comparative studies of lamivudine-zidovudine nanoparticles for the selective uptake by macrophages. *Curr Drug Deliv.* 2012;9(5):506-14. doi: 10.2174/156720 112802650707.

[121] Shegokar R, Singh KK. Stavudine entrapped lipid nanoparticles for targeting lymphatic HIV reservoirs. *Pharmazie.* 2011;66(4):264-71.

[122] Lahkar S, Kumar Das M. Surface modified kokum butter lipid nanoparticles for the brain targeted delivery of nevirapine. *J Microencapsul.* 2018;35(7-8):680-694. doi: 10.1080/02652048.2019.1573857.

[123] Desai J, Thakkar H. Effect of particle size on oral bioavailability of darunavir-loaded solid lipid nanoparticles. *J Microencapsul.* 2016;33(7):669-78. doi: 10.1080/02652048.2016.1245363.

[124] Jones E, Ojewole E, Kalhapure R, Govender T. In vitro comparative evaluation of monolayered multipolymeric films embedded with didanosine-loaded solid lipid nanoparticles: a potential buccal drug delivery system for ARV therapy. *Drug Dev Ind Pharm.* 2014;40(5):669-79. doi: 10.3109/03639045.2014.892957.

[125] Makwana V, Jain R, Patel K, Nivsarkar M, Joshi A. Solid lipid nanoparticles (SLN) of Efavirenz as lymph targeting drug delivery system: Elucidation of mechanism of uptake using chylomicron flow blocking approach. *Int J Pharm.* 2015;495(1): 439-46. doi: 10.1016/j.ijpharm.2015.09.014.

[126] Gupta S, Kesarla R, Chotai N, Misra A, Omri A. Systematic approach for the formulation and optimization of solid lipid nanoparticles of efavirenz by high pressure homogenization using design of experiments for brain targeting and enhanced bioavailability. *Biomed Res Int.* 2017; 2017:5984014. doi: 10.1155/2017/ 5984014.

[127] Alukda D, Sturgis T, Youan BC. Formulation of tenofovir-loaded functionalized solid lipid nanoparticles intended for HIV prevention. *J Pharm Sci.* 2011;100(8): 3345-56. doi: 10.1002/jps.22529.

[128] Lv Q, Yu A, Xi Y, Li H, Song Z, Cui J, Cao F, Zhai G. Development and evaluation of penciclovir-loaded solid lipid nanoparticles for topical delivery. *Int J Pharm.* 2009;372(1-2):191-8. doi: 10.1016/j.ijpharm.2009.01.014.

[129] Jain S, Mistry MA, Swarnakar NK. Enhanced dermal delivery of acyclovir using solid lipid nanoparticles. *Drug Deliv Transl Res.* 2011;1(5):395-406. doi: 10.1007/ s13346-011-0036-0.

[130] Kumar R, Sinha VR. Lipid nanocarrier: an efficient approach towards ocular delivery of hydrophilic drug (valacyclovir). *AAPS Pharm Sci Tech.* 2017;18(3): 884-94. doi: 10.1208/s12249-016-0575-2.

[131] Zhang XG, Miao J, Li MW, Jiang SP, Hu FQ, Du YZ. Solid lipid nanoparticles loading adefovir dipivoxil for antiviral therapy. *J Zhejiang Univ Sci B.* 2008;9(6): 506-10. doi: 10.1631/jzus.B0820047.

[132] Shi LL, Cao Y, Zhu XY, Cui JH, Cao QR. Optimization of process variables of zanamivir-loaded solid lipid nanoparticles and the prediction of their cellular transport in Caco-2 cell model. *Int J Pharm.* 2015;478(1):60-9. doi: 10.1016/j.ijpharm.2014.11.017.

[133] Cao Q, Wu H, Zhu L, Wu D, Zhu Y, Zhu Z, Cui J. Preparation and evaluation of zanamivir-loaded solid lipid nanoparticles. *J Control Release.* 2011;152 Suppl 1:e2-4. doi: 10.1016/j.jconrel.2011.08.085.

[134] Ren J, Zou M, Gao P, Wang Y, Cheng G. Tissue distribution of borneol-modified ganciclovir-loaded solid lipid nanoparticles in mice after intravenous administration. *Eur J Pharm Biopharm.* 2013;83(2):141-8. doi: 10.1016/j.ejpb.2012.10.018.

[135] Torgerson PR, Devleesschauwer B, Praet N, Speybroeck N, Willingham AL, Kasuga F, Rokni MB, Zhou XN, Fèvre EM, Sripa B, Gargouri N, Fürst T, Budke CM, Carabin H, Kirk MD, Angulo FJ, Havelaar A, de Silva N. world health organization estimates of the global and regional disease burden of 11 foodborne parasitic diseases, 2010: A data synthesis. *PLoS Med.* 2015;12(12):e1001920. doi: 10.1371/journal.pmed.1001920.

[136] Matthews KR. Controlling and coordinating development in vector-transmitted parasites. *Science.* 2011;331(6021):1149-53. doi: 10.1126/science.1198077.

[137] CDC, *Parasites.* https://www.cdc.gov/parasites/index.html (accessed 30 January 2020).

[138] Theel ES, Pritt BS. Parasites. In: Hayden RT, Wolk DM, Carroll KC, Tang Y (Eds.). *Diagnostic Microbiology of the Immunocompromised Host, ASM,* 2016, pp. 283-330. doi: 10.1128/9781555819040.ch18.

[139] Institute of Medicine (US) Forum on Microbial Threats. The causes and impacts of neglected tropical and zoonotic diseases: Opportunities for integrated intervention strategies. Washington (DC): National Academies Press (US); 2011. *Workshop Overview.* Available from: https://www.ncbi.nlm.nih.gov/books/NBK62526/.

[140] Andrade LN, Oliveira DML, Chaud MV, Alves TFR, Nery M, da Silva CF, Gonsalves JKC, Nunes RS, Corrêa CB, Amaral RG, Sanchez-Lopez E, Souto EB, Severino P. Praziquantel-solid lipid nanoparticles produced by supercritical carbon dioxide extraction: physicochemical characterization, release profile, and cytotoxicity. *Molecules.* 2019;24(21):3881. doi: 10.3390/molecules24213881.

[141] Adekiya TA, Kumar P, Kondiah PPD, Ubanako P, Choonara YE. *In vivo* evaluation of praziquantel-loaded solid lipid nanoparticles against *S. mansoni* infection in preclinical murine models. *Int J Mol Sci.* 2022;23(16):9485. doi: 10.3390/ijms23169485.

[142] Radwan A, El-Lakkany NM, William S, El-Feky GS, Al-Shorbagy MY, Saleh S, Botros S. A novel praziquantel solid lipid nanoparticle formulation shows enhanced bioavailability and antischistosomal efficacy against murine *S. mansoni* infection. *Parasit Vectors.* 2019;12(1):304. doi: 10.1186/s13071-019-3563-z.

[143] Xie S, Pan B, Wang M, Zhu L, Wang F, Dong Z, Wang X, Zhou W. Formulation, characterization and pharmacokinetics of praziquantel-loaded hydrogenated castor oil solid lipid nanoparticles. *Nanomedicine* (Lond). 20105(5):693-701. doi: 10.2217/nnm.10.42.

[144] de Souza AL, Andreani T, de Oliveira RN, Kiill CP, dos Santos FK, Allegretti SM, Chaud MV, Souto EB, Silva AM, Gremião MP. *In vitro* evaluation of permeation, toxicity and effect of praziquantel-loaded solid lipid nanoparticles against Schistosoma mansoni as a strategy to improve efficacy of the schistosomiasis treatment. *Int J Pharm.* 2014;463(1):31-7. doi: 10.1016/j.ijpharm.2013.12.022.

[145] Aminpour S, Rafiei A, Jelowdar A, Kouchak M. Evaluation of the protoscolicidal effects of albendazole and albendazole loaded solid lipid nanoparticles. *Iran J Parasitol.* 2019;14(1):127-35.

[146] Kohansal K, Rafiei A, Kalantari H, Jelowdar A, Salimi A, Rezaie A, Razi Jalali M. Nephrotoxicity of albendazole and albendazole loaded solid lipid nanoparticles in mice with experimental hydatidosis. *Adv Pharm Bull.* 2022;12(1):102-8. doi: 10.34172/apb.2022.011.

[147] Devi R, Jain A, Hurkat P, Jain SK. Dual drug delivery using lactic acid conjugated sln for effective management of neurocysticercosis. *Pharm Res.* 2015;32(10):3137-48. doi: 10.1007/s11095-015-1677-3.

[148] Permana AD, Tekko IA, McCrudden MTC, Anjani QK, Ramadon D, McCarthy HO, Donnelly RF. Solid lipid nanoparticle-based dissolving microneedles: A promising intradermal lymph targeting drug delivery system with potential for enhanced treatment of lymphatic filariasis. *J Control Release.* 2019;316:34-52. doi: 10.1016/j.jconrel.2019.10.004.

[149] Siram K, Chellan VR, Natarajan T, Krishnamoorthy B, Mohamed Ebrahim HR, Karanam V, Muthuswamy SS, Ranganathan HP. Solid lipid nanoparticles of diethylcarbamazine citrate for enhanced delivery to the lymphatics: in vitro and in vivo evaluation. *Expert Opin Drug Deliv.* 2014;11(9):1351-65. doi: 10.1517/17425247.2014.915310.

[150] Rehman MU, Khan MA, Khan WS, Shafique M, Khan M. Fabrication of Niclosamide loaded solid lipid nanoparticles: *in vitro* characterization and comparative *in vivo* evaluation. *Artif Cells Nanomed Biotechnol.* 2018;46(8):1926-34. doi: 10.1080/21691401.2017.1396996.

[151] Guo D, Dou D, Li X, Zhang Q, Bhutto ZA, Wang L. Ivermection-loaded solid lipid nanoparticles: preparation, characterisation, stability and transdermal behaviour. *Artif Cells Nanomed Biotechnol.* 2018;46(2):255-62. doi: 10.1080/21691401.2017.1307207.

[152] Aditya NP, Patankar S, Madhusudhan B, Murthy RS, Souto EB. Arthemeter-loaded lipid nanoparticles produced by modified thin-film hydration: Pharmacokinetics, toxicological and in vivo anti-malarial activity. *Eur J Pharm Sci.* 2010;40(5):448-55. doi: 10.1016/j.ejps.2010.05.007.

[153] Masiiwa WL, Gadaga LL. Intestinal permeability of artesunate-loaded solid lipid nanoparticles using the everted gut method. *J Drug Deliv.* 2018;2018:3021738. doi: 10.1155/2018/3021738.

[154] Omwoyo WN, Melariri P, Gathirwa JW, Oloo F, Mahanga GM, Kalombo L, Ogutu B, Swai H. Development, characterization and antimalarial efficacy of dihydroartemisinin loaded solid lipid nanoparticles. *Nanomedicine.* 2016;12(3): 801-9. doi: 10.1016/j.nano.2015.11.017.

[155] Muga JO, Gathirwa JW, Tukulula M, Jura WGZO. *In vitro* evaluation of chloroquine-loaded and heparin surface-functionalized solid lipid nanoparticles. *Malar J.* 2018;17(1):133. doi: 10.1186/s12936-018-2302-9.

[156] Omwoyo WN, Ogutu B, Oloo F, Swai H, Kalombo L, Melariri P, Mahanga GM, Gathirwa JW. Preparation, characterization, and optimization of primaquine-loaded solid lipid nanoparticles. *Int J Nanomedicine.* 2014;9:3865-74. doi: 10.21 47/IJN.S62630.

[157] Gupta Y, Jain A, Jain SK. Transferrin-conjugated solid lipid nanoparticles for enhanced delivery of quinine dihydrochloride to the brain. *J Pharm Pharmacol.* 2007;59(7):935-40. doi: 10.1211/jpp.59.7.0004.

[158] Khosravi M, Mohammad Rahimi H, Doroud D, Mirsamadi ES, Mirjalali H, Zali MR. In vitro Evaluation of mannosylated paromomycin-loaded solid lipid nanoparticles on acute toxoplasmosis. *Front Cell Infect Microbiol.* 2020;10:33. doi: 10.3389/fcimb.2020.00033.

[159] Heidari-Kharaji M, Taheri T, Doroud D, Habibzadeh S, Badirzadeh A, Rafati S. Enhanced paromomycin efficacy by solid lipid nanoparticle formulation against *Leishmania* in mice model. *Parasite Immunol.* 2016;38(10):599-608. doi: 10.11 11/pim.12340.

[160] Parvez S, Yadagiri G, Gedda MR, Singh A, Singh OP, Verma A, Sundar S, Mudavath SL. Modified solid lipid nanoparticles encapsulated with Amphotericin B and Paromomycin: an effective oral combination against experimental murine visceral leishmaniasis. *Sci Rep.* 2020;10(1):12243. doi: 10.1038/s41598-020-69 276-5.

[161] Singh A, Yadagiri G, Parvez S, Singh OP, Verma A, Sundar S, Mudavath SL. Formulation, characterization and in vitro anti-leishmanial evaluation of amphotericin B loaded solid lipid nanoparticles coated with vitamin B12-stearic acid conjugate. *Mater Sci Eng C Mater Biol Appl.* 2020;117:111279. doi: 10.10 16/j.msec.2020.111279.

[162] WHO, *Global Tuberculosis Report* 2020. https://apps.who.int/iris/bitstream/handle/10665/336069/9789240013131-eng.pdf (Accesed 02 February 2021).

[163] WHO, *Tuberculosis*. https://www.who.int/news-room/fact-sheets/detail/tuberculos is (Accesed 02 February 2021).

[164] Khatak S, Mehta M, Awasthi R, Paudel KR, Singh SK, Gulati M, Hansbro NG, Hansbro PM, Dua K, Dureja H. Solid lipid nanoparticles containing anti-tubercular drugs attenuate the *Mycobacterium marinum* infection. *Tuberculosis* (Edinb). 2020;125:102008. doi: 10.1016/j.tube.2020.102008.

[165] Pandey R, Sharma S, Khuller GK. Oral solid lipid nanoparticle-based antitubercular chemotherapy. *Tuberculosis* (Edinb). 2005;85(5-6):415-20. doi: 10. 1016/j.tube.2005.08.009.

[166] Bhandari R, Kaur IP. Pharmacokinetics, tissue distribution and relative bioavailability of isoniazid-solid lipid nanoparticles. *Int J Pharm.* 2013;441(1-2):202-12. doi: 10.1016/j.ijpharm.2012.11.042.

[167] Vieira ACC, Chaves LL, Pinheiro M, Lima SAC, Ferreira D, Sarmento B, Reis S. Mannosylated solid lipid nanoparticles for the selective delivery of rifampicin to macrophages. *Artif Cells Nanomed Biotechnol.* 2018;46(sup1):653-63. doi: 10.1080/21691401.2018.1434186.

[168] Vieira ACC, Chaves LL, Pinheiro S, Pinto S, Pinheiro M, Lima SC, Ferreira D, Sarmento B, Reis S. Mucoadhesive chitosan-coated solid lipid nanoparticles for better management of tuberculosis. *Int J Pharm.* 2018;536(1):478-85. doi: 10.1016/j.ijpharm.2017.11.071.

[169] Costa A, Sarmento B, Seabra V. Mannose-functionalized solid lipid nanoparticles are effective in targeting alveolar macrophages. *Eur J Pharm Sci.* 2018;114:103-113. doi: 10.1016/j.ejps.2017.12.006.

[170] Nemati E, Mokhtarzadeh A, Panahi-Azar V, Mohammadi A, Hamishehkar H, Mesgari-Abbasi M, Ezzati Nazhad Dolatabadi J, de la Guardia M. Ethambutol-Loaded Solid Lipid Nanoparticles as Dry Powder Inhalable Formulation for Tuberculosis Therapy. *AAPS Pharm Sci Tech.* 2019;20(3):120. doi: 10.1208/s12249-019-1334-y.

[171] Kumar M, Kakkar V, Mishra AK, Chuttani K, Kaur IP. Intranasal delivery of streptomycin sulfate (STRS) loaded solid lipid nanoparticles to brain and blood. *Int J Pharm.* 2014;461(1-2):223-33. doi: 10.1016/j.ijpharm.2013.11.038.

[172] Chetoni P, Burgalassi S, Monti D, Tampucci S, Tullio V, Cuffini AM, Muntoni E, Spagnolo R, Zara GP, Cavalli R. Solid lipid nanoparticles as promising tool for intraocular tobramycin delivery: Pharmacokinetic studies on rabbits. *Eur J Pharm Biopharm.* 2016;109:214-223. doi: 10.1016/j.ejpb.2016.10.006.

[173] Nair AB, Shah J, Al-Dhubiab BE, Jacob S, Patel SS, Venugopala KN, Morsy MA, Gupta S, Attimarad M, Sreeharsha N, Shinu P. Clarithromycin solid lipid nanoparticles for topical ocular therapy: optimization, evaluation and *in vivo* studies. *Pharmaceutics.* 2021;13(4):523. doi: 10.3390/pharmaceutics13040523.

[174] Sharma M, Gupta N, Gupta S. Implications of designing clarithromycin loaded solid lipid nanoparticles on its pharmacokinetics, antibacterial activity and safety. *RSC Adv.* 2016; doi: 10.1039/C6RA12841F.

[175] Dong Z, Xie S, Zhu L, Wang Y, Wang X, Zhou W. Preparation and *in vitro, in vivo* evaluations of norfloxacin-loaded solid lipid nanopartices for oral delivery. *Drug Deliv.* 2011;18(6):441-50. doi: 10.3109/10717544.2011.577109.

[176] Bhattacharyya S, Reddy P. Effect of surfactant on azithromycin dihydrate loaded stearic acid solid lipid nanoparticles. *Turk J Pharm Sci.* 2019;16(4):425-31. doi: 10.4274/tjps.galenos.2018.82160.

[177] Pignatello R, Leonardi A, Fuochi V, Petronio Petronio G, Greco AS, Furneri PM. A method for efficient loading of ciprofloxacin hydrochloride in cationic solid lipid nanoparticles: Formulation and microbiological evaluation. *Nanomaterials.* 2018; 8(5): 304.

[178] Hosseini SM, Farmany A, Abbasalipourkabir R, Soleimani Asl S, Nourian A, Arabestani MR. Doxycycline-encapsulated solid lipid nanoparticles for the

enhanced antibacterial potential to treat the chronic brucellosis and preventing its relapse: *in vivo* study. *Ann Clin Microbiol Antimicrob.* 2019;18(1):33. doi: 10.1186/s12941-019-0333-x.

[179] Hosseini SM, Abbasalipourkabir R, Jalilian FA, Asl SS, Farmany A, Roshanaei G, Arabestani MR. Doxycycline-encapsulated solid lipid nanoparticles as promising tool against *Brucella melitensis* enclosed in macrophage: a pharmacodynamics study on J774A.1 cell line. *Antimicrob Resist Infect Control.* 2019;8:62. doi: 10.1186/s13756-019-0504-8.

[180] Severino P, Chaud MV, Shimojo A, Antonini D, Lancelloti M, Santana MH, Souto EB. Sodium alginate-cross-linked polymyxin B sulphate-loaded solid lipid nanoparticles: Antibiotic resistance tests and HaCat and NIH/3T3 cell viability studies. *Colloids Surf B Biointerfaces.* 2015;129:191-7. doi: 10.1016/j.colsurfb. 2015.03.049.

[181] Severino P, Silveira EF, Loureiro K, Chaud MV, Antonini D, Lancellotti M, Sarmento VH, da Silva CF, Santana MHA, Souto EB. Antimicrobial activity of polymyxin-loaded solid lipid nanoparticles (PLX-SLN): Characterization of physicochemical properties and in vitro efficacy. *Eur J Pharm Sci.* 2017;106:177-84. doi: 10.1016/j.ejps.2017.05.063.

[182] Aldawsari HM, Hosny KM. Solid lipid nanoparticles of Vancomycin loaded with Ellagic acid as a tool for overcoming nephrotoxic side effects: preparation, characterization, and nephrotoxicity evaluation. *J Drug Deliv Sci Technol.* 2018; 45: 76-80.

[183] Ghanem A, Healey R, Adly FG. Current trends in separation of plasmid DNA vaccines: a review. *Anal Chim Acta.* 2013;760:1-15. doi: 10.1016/j.aca.2012.11. 006.

[184] Malone RW, Felgner PL, Verma IM. Cationic liposome-mediated RNA transfection. *Proc Natl Acad Sci U S A.* 1989;86(16):6077-81. doi: 10.1073/pnas. 86.16.6077.

[185] Thi TTH, Suys EJA, Lee JS, Nguyen DH, Park KD, Truong NP. Lipid-Based Nanoparticles in the Clinic and Clinical Trials: From Cancer Nanomedicine to COVID-19 Vaccines. *Vaccines* (Basel). 2021 Apr 8;9(4):359. doi: 10.3390/vac cines9040359.

[186] Pardi N, Hogan MJ, Porter FW, Weissman D. mRNA vaccines - a new era in vaccinology. *Nat Rev Drug Discov.* 2018;17(4):261-279. doi: 10.1038/nrd.2017. 243.

[187] Jackson LA, Anderson EJ, Rouphael NG, Roberts PC, Makhene M, Coler RN, McCullough MP, Chappell JD, Denison MR, Stevens LJ, Pruijssers AJ, McDermott A, Flach B, Doria-Rose NA, Corbett KS, Morabito KM, O'Dell S, Schmidt SD, Swanson PA 2nd, Padilla M, Mascola JR, Neuzil KM, Bennett H, Sun W, Peters E, Makowski M, Albert J, Cross K, Buchanan W, Pikaart-Tautges R, Ledgerwood JE, Graham BS, Beigel JH; mRNA-1273 Study Group. An mRNA Vaccine against SARS-CoV-2 - Preliminary Report. *N Engl J Med.* 2020;383(20): 1920-1931. doi: 10.1056/NEJMoa2022483.

[188] Chira S, Jackson CS, Oprea I, Ozturk F, Pepper MS, Diaconu I, Braicu C, Raduly LZ, Calin GA, Berindan-Neagoe I. Progresses towards safe and efficient gene

therapy vectors. *Oncotarget.* 2015;6(31):30675-703. doi: 10.18632/oncotarget.5169.

[189] Ramamoorth M, Narvekar A. Non viral vectors in gene therapy- an overview. *J Clin Diagn Res.* 2015;9(1):GE01-6. doi: 10.7860/JCDR/2015/10443.5394.

[190] Foldvari M, Chen DW, Nafissi N, Calderon D, Narsineni L, Rafiee A. Non-viral gene therapy: Gains and challenges of non-invasive administration methods. *J Control Release.* 2016;240:165-190. doi: 10.1016/j.jconrel.2015.12.012.

[191] del Pozo-Rodríguez A, Delgado D, Solinís MA, Gascón AR, Pedraz JL. Solid lipid nanoparticles: formulation factors affecting cell transfection capacity. *Int J Pharm.* 2007;339(1-2):261-8. doi: 10.1016/j.ijpharm.2007.03.015.

[192] Mansouri S, Lavigne P, Corsi K, Benderdour M, Beaumont E, Fernandes JC. Chitosan-DNA nanoparticles as non-viral vectors in gene therapy: strategies to improve transfection efficacy. *Eur J Pharm Biopharm.* 2004;57(1):1-8. doi: 10.1016/s0939-6411(03)00155-3.

[193] Han Z, Conley SM, Makkia R, Guo J, Cooper MJ, Naash MI. Comparative analysis of DNA nanoparticles and AAVs for ocular gene delivery. *PLoS One.* 2012;7(12): e52189. doi: 10.1371/journal.pone.0052189.

[194] Slivac I, Guay D, Mangion M, Champeil J, Gaillet B. Non-viral nucleic acid delivery methods. *Expert Opin Biol Ther.* 2017;17(1):105-18. doi: 10.1080/14712598.2017.1248941.

[195] Rivest V, Phivilay A, Julien C, Bélanger S, Tremblay C, Emond V, Calon F. Novel liposomal formulation for targeted gene delivery. *Pharm Res.* 2007;24(5):981-90. doi: 10.1007/s11095-006-9224-x.

[196] Masotti A, Mossa G, Cametti C, Ortaggi G, Bianco A, Grosso ND, Malizia D, Esposito C. Comparison of different commercially available cationic liposome-DNA lipoplexes: Parameters influencing toxicity and transfection efficiency. *Colloids Surf B Biointerfaces.* 2009;68(2):136-44. doi: 10.1016/j.colsurfb.2008.09.017.

[197] Martini E, Fattal E, de Oliveira MC, Teixeira H. Effect of cationic lipid composition on properties of oligonucleotide/emulsion complexes: Physico-chemical and release studies. *Int J Pharm.* 2008;352(1-2):280-6. doi: 10.1016/j.ijpharm.2007.10.032.

[198] Hassett KJ, Benenato KE, Jacquinet E, Lee A, Woods A, Yuzhakov O, Himansu S, Deterling J, Geilich BM, Ketova T, Mihai C, Lynn A, McFadyen I, Moore MJ, Senn JJ, Stanton MG, Almarsson Ö, Ciaramella G, Brito LA. Optimization of Lipid Nanoparticles for Intramuscular Administration of mRNA Vaccines. *Mol Ther Nucleic Acids.* 2019;15:1-11. doi: 10.1016/j.omtn.2019.01.013.

[199] Penumarthi A, Parashar D, Abraham A, Dekiwadia C, Macreadie I, Shukla R, Smooker P. Solid lipid nanoparticles mediate non-viral delivery of plasmid DNA to dendritic cells. *J Nanoparticle Res.* 2017;19(210):1–10. doi: 10.1007/s11051-017-3902-y.

[200] Kim HR, Kim IK, Bae KH, Lee SH, Lee Y, Park TG. Cationic solid lipid nanoparticles reconstituted from low density lipoprotein components for delivery of siRNA. *Mol Pharm.* 2008;5(4):622-31. doi: 10.1021/mp8000233.

[201] Asasutjarit R, Lorenzen SI, Sirivichayakul S, Ruxrungtham K, Ruktanonchai U, Ritthidej GC. Effect of solid lipid nanoparticles formulation compositions on their size, zeta potential and potential for in vitro pHIS-HIV-hugag transfection. *Pharm Res.* 2007;24(6):1098-107. doi: 10.1007/s11095-007-9234-3.

[202] Li S, Yang Y, Lin X, Li Z, Ma G, Su Z, Zhang S. Biocompatible cationic solid lipid nanoparticles as adjuvants effectively improve humoral and T cell immune response of foot and mouth disease vaccines. *Vaccine.* 2020;38(11):2478-2486. doi: 10.1016/j.vaccine.2020.02.004.

[203] Fàbregas A, Prieto-Sánchez S, Suñé-Pou M, Boyero-Corral S, Ticó JR, García-Montoya E, Pérez-Lozano P, Miñarro M, Suñé-Negre JM, Hernández-Munain C, Suñé C. Improved formulation of cationic solid lipid nanoparticles displays cellular uptake and biological activity of nucleic acids. *Int J Pharm.* 2017;516(1-2):39-44. doi: 10.1016/j.ijpharm.2016.11.026.

[204] Suñé-Pou M, Prieto-Sánchez S, El Yousfi Y, Boyero-Corral S, Nardi-Ricart A, Nofrerias-Roig I, Pérez-Lozano P, García-Montoya E, Miñarro-Carmona M, Ticó JR, Suñé-Negre JM, Hernández-Munain C, Suñé C. Cholesteryl oleate-loaded cationic solid lipid nanoparticles as carriers for efficient gene-silencing therapy. *Int J Nanomedicine.* 2018;13:3223-3233. doi: 10.2147/IJN.S158884.

[205] Apaolaza PS, Del Pozo-Rodríguez A, Solinís MA, Rodríguez JM, Friedrich U, Torrecilla J, Weber BH, Rodríguez-Gascón A. Structural recovery of the retina in a retinoschisin-deficient mouse after gene replacement therapy by solid lipid nanoparticles. *Biomaterials.* 2016;90:40-9. doi: 10.1016/j.biomaterials.2016.03.00 4.

[206] Francis JE, Skakic I, Dekiwadia C, Shukla R, Taki AC, Walduck A, Smooker PM. Solid Lipid Nanoparticle Carrier Platform Containing Synthetic TLR4 Agonist Mediates Non-Viral DNA Vaccine Delivery. *Vaccines* (Basel). 2020;8(3):551. doi: 10.3390/vaccines8030551.

[207] Almeida AJ, Souto E. Solid lipid nanoparticles as a drug delivery system for peptides and proteins. *Adv Drug Deliv Rev.* 2007;59(6):478-90. doi: 10.1016/j.ad dr.2007.04.007.

[208] Mishra H, Mishra D, Mishra PK, Nahar M, Dubey V, Jain NK. Evaluation of solid lipid nanoparticles as carriers for delivery of hepatitis B surface antigen for vaccination using subcutaneous route. *J Pharm Pharm Sci.* 2010;13(4):495-509. doi: 10.18433/j3xk53.

[209] Saraf S, Sahoo RN, Jain S, Mallick S. M-cell Targeting Acid-resistant Oral Vaccine Delivery for Immunization Against Hepatitis B Infection Using Cationic *Solid Lipid Nanoparticles.* 2021. doi: https://doi.org/10.21203/rs.3.rs-904521/v1.

[210] del Pozo-Rodríguez A, Delgado D, Solinís MA, Gascón AR, Pedraz JL. Solid lipid nanoparticles: formulation factors affecting cell transfection capacity. *Int J Pharm.* 2007;339(1-2):261-8. doi: 10.1016/j.ijpharm.2007.03.015.

[211] Pardi N, Hogan MJ, Porter FW, Weissman D. mRNA vaccines—A new era in vaccinology. *Nat. Rev. Drug Discov.* 2018;17:261–279. doi: 10.1038/nrd.2017.24 3.

[212] Vogel, AB, Lambert, L, Kinnear, E, Busse, D, Erbar, S, Reuter, KC, Wicke, L, Perkovic, M, Beissert, T, Haas, H, Reece, ST, Sahin, U, & Tregoning, JS. Self-

Amplifying RNA Vaccines Give Equivalent Protection against Influenza to mRNA Vaccines but at Much Lower Doses. *Mol. Ther.* 2018;26:446–455. doi: 10.1016/j.ymthe.2017.11.017.

[213] Magini D, Giovani C, Mangiavacchi S, Maccari S, Cecchi R, Ulmer JB, De Gregorio E, Geall AJ, Brazzoli M, Bertholet S. Self-Amplifying mRNA Vaccines Expressing Multiple Conserved Influenza Antigens Confer Protection against Homologous and Heterosubtypic Viral Challenge. *PLoS ONE.* 2016;11:e0161193. doi: 10.1371/journal.pone.0161193.

[214] Anderluzzi G, Lou G, Gallorini S, Brazzoli M, Johnson R, O'Hagan DT, Baudner BC, Perrie Y. Investigating the Impact of Delivery System Design on the Efficacy of Self-Amplifying RNA Vaccines. *Vaccines* (Basel). 2020;8(2):212. doi: 10.3390/vaccines8020212.

[215] Doroud D, Zahedifard F, Vatanara A, Najafabadi AR, Taslimi Y, Vahabpour R, Torkashvand F, Vaziri B, Rafati S. Delivery of a cocktail DNA vaccine encoding cysteine proteinases type I, II and III with solid lipid nanoparticles potentiate protective immunity against *Leishmania major* infection. *J Control Release.* 2011; 153(2):154-62. doi: 10.1016/j.jconrel.2011.04.011.

[216] Saljoughian N, Zahedifard F, Doroud D, Doustdari F, Vasei M, Papadopoulou B, Rafati S. Cationic solid-lipid nanoparticles are as efficient as electroporation in DNA vaccination against visceral leishmaniasis in mice. *Parasite Immunol.* 2013;35(12):397-408. doi: 10.1111/pim.12042.

Chapter 2

An Agent-Based Model of Infectious Diseases That Incorporates the Roles of Immune Cells and Antibodies

Shigeaki Ogibayashi
Chiba Institute of Technology, Chiba, Japan

Abstract

In this study, an agent-based infection model focusing on recovery process modeling was constructed, and the following results were obtained. The present model well reproduced the qualitative features of the chronological pattern in the numbers of newly infected, newly recovered, and total infected agents observed in the real world. The factors of the model that are indispensable for reproducing the actual pandemic are the roles of fever and antibodies, which increase the upper limit of the rate of virus replication for pandemic convergence.

The role of fever is modeled as the effect of immunity increasing with an increasing number of viruses, and the role of antibodies is modeled as antibodies emerging when the immunity is insufficient to keep up with virus replication. The critical factor determining whether pandemic convergence occurs is whether the system includes severely infected agents whose immune response cannot keep up with the virus replication rate. Such severely infected agents are characterized by a high body temperature and a massive number of viruses. To control infection spread, it is essential to identify infected individuals, especially severely infected ones, and isolate them from the system. Measuring body temperature is effective in identifying severely infected individuals, rather than PCR tests, because fever is a sign of being infected and also provides information about the severity of infection, while PCR tests provide information only in a dichotomous positive/negative format.

In: Infectious Diseases
Editor: Yvette S. Brewer
ISBN: 979-8-88697-657-1

To overcome the pandemic while minimizing the economic impact, it is effective to identify and isolate infected individuals by monitoring body temperature and refusing entry of those infected at national borders, such as airports, and also in densely populated places. It is also effective for individuals to determine their own infection status by monitoring their own body temperature. Wearing masks and providing ventilation in densely populated spaces are also effective because they decrease the number of viruses at the time of infection.

Keywords: agent-based model, infectious disease, SARS-CoV-2, immune cell, antibody, fever, virus, viral particle, pandemic, convergence, infection, recovery

Introduction

Since the novel coronavirus, namely, Severe Acute Respiratory Syndrome Coronavirus 2 (SARS-CoV-2), was first discovered in December 2019 in China, it has spread worldwide and the number of infections is still increasing in most countries. Although restrictions on movement have led to the number of infections reaching a low level as of July 10, 2020 (Worldmeter/coronavirus_updates, 2020), many countries are beginning to ease the tight control of social activity to help their economies recover, despite worries about the emergence of another wave of this pandemic.

Many mathematical models for forecasting the emergence of a pandemic were constructed long before the ongoing pandemic began (Bailey, N. T. J., 1975: Li, M. Y., 2019: Britton, T. and Ball, F., 2019: Marchuk, G. I., 2019, Anderson, R. M. and May, R. M., 1991: Vynnycky, E. and White, R., 2010). Most of these models are system-dynamics models such as the SIR model and SIER model, consisting of a set of equations to be solved simultaneously. The infection and recovery process is modeled simply by introducing a set of parameters representing the probability of a healthy person being infected and an infected person recovering. However, these equation-based models have the fatal flaw of being unable to describe the complex interactions among heterogeneous agents that are the essential cause of infectious disease propagation. Furthermore, such models do not provide knowledge on the factors influencing recovery or the occurrence of another wave of the pandemic because they do not describe the post-infection recovery process from the bottom up.

Agent-based modeling (ABM) is a modeling method suitable for describing the heterogeneity of the behaviors of agents (Wilensky, U. and

White, R., 2010: Epstein, J. M. and Axtell, R., 1995). In ABM, we construct an artificial society on a computer that mimics the real world, aiming to reproduce various social phenomena caused by the behaviors and interactions of agents from the bottom up. Thus, ABM is an effective way to understand the underlying mechanism and solve economic and social problems (Epstein, J. M. and Axtell, R., 1995: Ogibayashi, S. and Takashima, K., 2017: Ogibayashi, S. and Takashima, K., 2019: Ogibayashi, S. and Shinagawa, K., 2020). ABM has various advantageous features, such as being able to deal with heterogeneity and discrete phenomena (Wilensky, U. and White, R., 2010), the essential advantageous characteristic of ABM is that it is a bottom-up modeling method.

Because social phenomena emerge due to humans' actions and interactions, we can use ABM to construct an artificial society that works according to the same principles as the real world. Notably, a model can work in this way only when that model is entirely bottom-up without using any aggregate-variable-related assumptions. Moreover, the types of agents and their behavioral rules and the relevant variables, that is, the system structure, must be as realistic as possible to reflect micro-level phenomena and thereby reproduce the macro-phenomena (Ogibayashi, S. and Takashima, K., 2017: Ogibayashi, S. and Takashima, K., 2019: Ogibayashi, S. and Shinagawa, K., 2020).

Although ABM has also been applied to diseases (Perez, L. and Dragicevic, S., 2009: Li, Y. et al., 2016: Tuomisto, J. T. et al., 2020: Rockett, R. J. et al., 2020), most of the resulting models are not fully bottom-up in that they employ aggregate-variable-related assumptions. In a few cases where the applied ABM was entirely bottom-up regarding the spatial interaction among agents, the post-infection recovery process was not modeled from the bottom-up in that infected agents were assumed to become immune at a specific period after infection and never be infected again (Perez, L. and Dragicevic, S., 2009). Thus, although models of this type can mimic the spatial interactions among agents that cause infection, they cannot reproduce the specific behaviors that increase or decrease the numbers of newly infected, newly recovered, and total infected persons without using macroscopic assumptions. Moreover, such models cannot predict the emergence of another wave of a pandemic after the easing of regulations concerning social movement.

According to statistical data (Worldmeter/coronavirus_updates, 2020), the numbers of total infected, newly infected, and newly cured persons in the pandemic peaked at different periods. Conventional models cannot explain these features without using macroscopic assumptions, neither the equation-based model nor the ABM model.

According to medical findings, when a person is infected, the virus enters the host's body and replicates, increasing the number of viruses. Regarding the function of immune cells and antibodies, it is well known (Eden, D., 2020) that immune cells are the first to attack the virus, followed by antibodies. Antibodies emerge after a certain period, joining the fight against the virus. The effect of fever is also well known (Shu, T., 2020). When viruses enter the host's body, they are attacked by the immune system and reduced in number, while they increase due to replication. If the rate at which they are reduced in number is exceeded by their replication speed, the host's body temperature may rise so that the effect of the immune system can keep up with the replication rate of viruses. According to the literature (Shu, T., 2020), an increase in body temperature by 1°C increases the intensity of the immune response by several fold. Thus, the host's body temperature keeps rising after infection until it peaks, after which it declines in line with the host's recovery. If the effect of immune cells along with fever is insufficient to achieve the host's recovery, antibodies emerge, which enhance the effect of the immune system.

Based on these medical findings, the fundamental factor that characterizes the infectious state is the virus, and the essential factors that characterize the recovery process are immune cells and antibodies. However, few previously reported epidemic models take these micro-factors into account. Against this background, the present research developed an agent-based model that incorporates the roles of immune cells and antibodies and the number of viruses, and compared the resulting data with real-world statistical data. The underlying mechanism for the spread of infection and convergence, and the conditions for balancing infection control and economic growth, are discussed.

The Model

Model Outline

This model considers the roles of immune cells and antibodies and the number of viruses. The interactions among agents are simplified, assuming random movement of agents.

In this model, the human agent is the only object that moves randomly in the two-dimensional space of 1 km^2 every period. The number of human agents is assumed to be 2000, and their initial positions in the two-dimensional space are assigned randomly for each agent. The distance and direction of movement are assigned in every period by a uniform random number, as given in Table 1. One of the individual humans is initially the infected agent, possessing many viruses, that is, viral particles, the number of which is an attribute variable. An agent is assumed to meet with another agent to become a neighbor when located within a critical distance, which is assumed to be 5 m. The infected human is assumed to release some of the viruses in every period at a predetermined virus-releasing rate in the form of a cough or other means. Thus, any agent who meets an infected neighbor receives a portion of the released viruses at a predetermined virus-absorbing rate, becoming a newly infected agent. A decrease in the virus-absorbing rate corresponds to the wearing of masks or face shields in the real world. The increasing number of viruses transferred from an infected agent to a healthy individual in each period is assumed as given by Equation (1).

$$\Delta N^{i}_{Infected}(t) = \sum_{j \in neighbors} N^{j}_{VP}(t) * Rate^{j}_{Release} * Rate^{i}_{absorb}$$

where, $\Delta N^{i}_{Infected}(t)$: *number of viruses of agent i transferred from neighbor agents at the time t*

$N_{VP}^{j}(t)$: *number of viruses of agent j at the time t*

$Rate^{j}_{Release}$: *virus releasing rate of agent j*

$Rate^{i}_{absorb}$: *virus absorbing rate of agent i*

(1)

If an agent is infected, immune cells attack the viruses at every time step, reducing their number at a predetermined virus attack rate of immune cells or antibodies. The decreasing number of viruses in each period at time t is assumed to be proportional to the number of viruses, as given by Equation (2). This assumption stems from the knowledge that, when the immune response cannot keep up with the speed of replication of the viruses, the host's body temperature rises, which increases the immune response. Here, the virus attack rate is assumed to be higher if antibodies are present. Antibodies are assumed to emerge that attack the viruses at a higher rate than that of immune cells, after a predetermined antibody-emerging period, if the agent's viral particles exceed a particular threshold. This threshold of the number of viruses required for antibody emergence is assumed to be the product of the number of viruses and the predetermined minimum-virus-count-multiple. The conditions required for the emergence of antibodies are assumed based on Equation (3).

For comparison, an additional series of experiments in which the right side of equation (2) is assumed to be a constant value was also conducted to better understand the roles of immune cells and antibodies in pandemic convergence. The constant value is assumed to be a constant multiple of the virus attack rate of immune cells or antibodies.

$$\Delta N^{i}{}_{VP}(t) = N^{i}{}_{VP}(t) * Rate^{i}{}_{attack}$$
$$\text{where, } \Delta N^{i}{}_{VP}(t): \textit{Decreasing increment of the number of viruses during the time stept}$$
$$Rate^{i}{}_{attack} = \textit{Virus attack rate of immune cells or antibodies} \tag{2}$$

$$t - t^{i}{}_{infected} > t^{i}{}_{antibody\_emerging} \quad \text{and} \quad N^{i}{}_{VP}(t) > N^{i}{}_{VP}(t^{i}{}_{infected}) * Multiple^{i}{}_{antibody\_emergence}$$
$$\text{where, } t: \textit{Current time}, \quad t^{i}{}_{infected}: \textit{Time of infection of agent i}$$
$$t^{i}{}_{antibody\_emerging}: \textit{Elapsed period for antibody emergence of agent i after infection}$$
$$Multiple^{i}{}_{antibody\_emergence}: \textit{Virus count multiple for antibody emergence} \tag{3}$$

The resultant viruses are assumed to multiply, increasing in number, due to viral replication at a predetermined virus replication rate. The virus replication rate represents the increase in the number of viruses per time step and is assumed to be constant during the calculation. Thus, the number of viruses is redefined at every time step according to Equation (4).

$$N^{i}{}_{VP}(t+1) = (1 - Rate^{i}{}_{Release} - Rate^{i}{}_{attack}) * N^{i}{}_{VP}(t) * Rate_{growth} + \Delta N^{i}{}_{Infected}(t)$$
$$\text{where, } Rate_{Release}: \textit{virus releasing rate of agent i}$$
$$Rate_{attack}: \textit{Virus attack rate of immune cells or antibodies of agent i}$$
$$Rate_{growth}: \textit{Virus replication rate defined as a constant value}$$
$$\Delta N^{i}{}_{Infected}(t): \textit{Increasing incerment of the number of viruses due to infection} \tag{4}$$

When the number of viruses of an agent becomes smaller than the critical lower limit, it is assumed to be zero as given by Equation (5); at this time, the agent state changes from infected to recovered, being classified as newly recovered. Here, the number of viruses is an arbitrary unit, so it could be below 1 in the present model.

$$N^{i}_{VP}(t) = 0,\ if\ N^{i}_{VP}(t) < N^{i}_{\min}$$
$$where,\ N^{i}_{\min} : n_{limit} * virus\ releasing\ rate * virus\ absorbing\ rate$$
$$n_{limit} : Critical\ value\ for\ zero\ viruses\ assumed\ as\ 10^{-9} \quad (5)$$

The attribute variables of agents and parameter values are presented in Table 1, where the variables that are defined by a uniform random number are agent-specific variables.

The present model does not incorporate agent death because it requires a massive population and thus the calculation time needed becomes too large. Moreover, the death rate is so low compared with the infection rate that it is not an essential factor in the mechanism of infection spread and convergence. Therefore, all of the infected agents finally recover in this model unless the virus replication rate is assumed to be too high.

Table 1. Attribute variables of agents and parameter values

Variables	Initial value or definition
Number of agents	2000
Area of network system	1000×1000
Maximum distance of agent's move	100,200
Critical distance for infection	5
Initial number of the infected	1
Number of viruses hold by the infected initially	5000×100 (arbitrary unit)
Virus replication rate	1.4,1.6,1.8,2.0
Virus attack rate by immune cells	0.3±0.1 uniform random number
Virus attack rate by antibodies	0.5±0.1 uniform random number
Virus-count multiple for antibody emergence	0.5±0.2 uniform random number
Elapsed period after infection for antibody emergence	7±2 uniform random number
Minimum number of viruses, below which number of viruses is assumed zero	10e-9 (arbitrary unit)
Virus releasing rate	0.1±0.05 uniform random number
Virus absorbing rate	0.1±0.05 uniform random number
Position (x, y) in the two-dimensional space	Defined at every step
Distance of agent's move	[0, maximum distance] uniform random number
Direction of agent's move	[0, 2π] uniform random number
Agent in the neighbor	Defined at every step
Number of viruses of each agent	Calculated at every step

The model is programmed by the author, using C++ with object-oriented programming. The fundamental classes used in the model are "Human," which moves randomly, "Human Aggregator" which manages the creation and state of "Human," "Germ," which is held by a Human class and responsible for the calculation of virus-related variables, and "Network," which manages the position of Humans and is responsible for the calculation of infection among agents. These classes refer to infection-related variables, such as the number of viruses and the distance between agents.

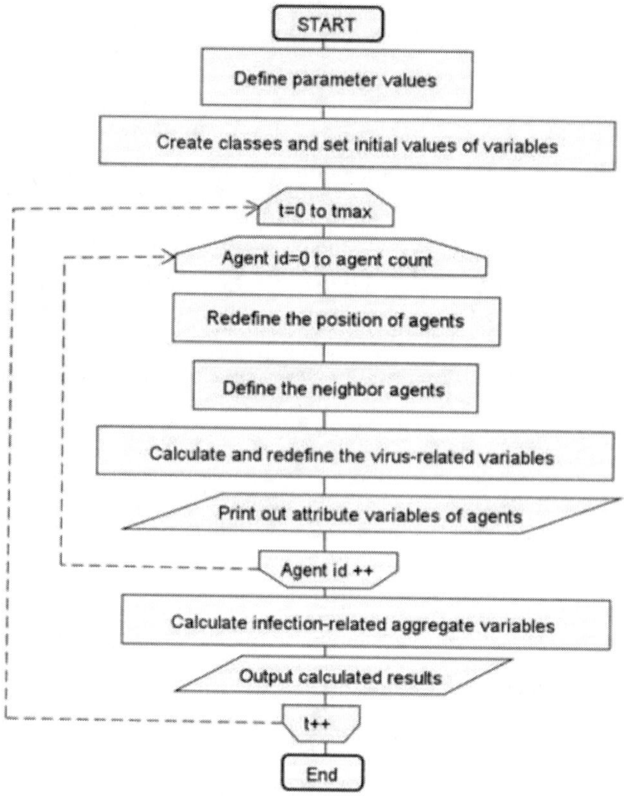

Figure 1. The flowchart of the calculation.

The calculation is processed according to the following steps. A flowchart of the calculation is presented in Figure 1.

a) Define parameter values.

b) Create various class objects and set initial values for the variables.
c) Repeat the following steps until the maximum time step is reached.
   i) For each agent, redefine the agent's position, define the neighbor agent, calculate the change in the number of viruses, and output the agent's attribute variables. The agent's attribute variables include the number of viruses transferred from infected agents at the time of new infection, the decrease in the number of viruses due to the role of immune cells or antibodies, the increase in the number of viruses due to virus replication, and various state variables.
   ii) Calculate aggregate variables, such as the numbers of infected agents and recovered agents and output the results.

Experimental Conditions

Analysis Items at Each Time Step

The characteristic variables calculated at every time step are divided into agent's attribute variables and state variables of the system and given in Table 2.

Table 2. Characteristic variables calculated at every time step

1. Agent's attributes variables
Number of viruses
Position in the two-dimensional space
Agents as objects located in the neighbor
Number of infected or uninfected neighbors
Number of viruses increased due to infection
Infection-related state variables
Uninfected, Infected and recovered with or without antibodies
2. State variables of the network system
Average numbers of neighbors, infected neighbors and uninfected neighbors
Number of infected agents
Number of newly infected agents
Number of newly recovered agents
Number of recovered agents with antibodies
Number of recovered agents without antibodies
Number of viruses in the system which is the sum of each agent's viruses.

The former variables include agents as objects located among neighbors, which are responsible for the mutual infection and determined based on the distance among agents in the two-dimensional space. The latter variables include the numbers of infected agents, newly infected agents, and newly recovered agents with or without antibodies. The changes in the calculated state variables over time were compared with the statistical data available in the real world.

Experimental Conditions

The influence of the following factors on the abovementioned variables was analyzed: 1) virus replication rate, 2) maximum traveling distance, 3) virus-absorbing rate (accounting for mask use), 4) implementation and relaxation of restrictions on agent movement that include temporary regulation of the distance that can be traveled with or without reducing the virus-absorbing rate, and 5) existence of antibodies.

Calculated Results

Fundamental Behavior during Infection and Recovery

This section describes the fundamental behavior of infection and recovery in the case without any countermeasures against disease. Here, as given by Equation (2), the decrease of each agent's number of viruses per time step due to the effect of immunity is assumed to be proportional to the number of viruses at each time step. This assumption corresponds to the development of a fever after infection in the real world, where the effect of immunity increases with an increase in the body temperature. Furthermore, the maximum distance of movement, the average value of the virus-absorbing rate, and the average values of the virus attack rates of immune cells and antibodies are each assumed to be constant. Please note that the particular attributes of each agent are heterogeneous, as given in Table 1.

Effect of Virus Replication Rate on the Numbers of Infected and Recovered Agents

Figure 2 shows the changes in the number of infected agents when the virus replication rate is changed from 1.4 to 2.0. The number of infected agents is represented as the percentage of the total population. When the virus replication rate is between 1.4 and 1.8, the number of infected agents increases, peaks, then decreases, ending the pandemic. In such cases, the virus replication rate is not too large compared with the virus attack rate of immune cells or antibodies. By contrast, when the virus replication rate is too large, such as 2.0, the entire population is eventually infected, and the pandemic does not end. When the virus replication rate is too low compared with the virus attack rate, the infection scale becomes too small to be called a pandemic. In the present model, the cases where the virus replication rate is between 1.4 and 1.8 correspond to situations observed in the real world; thus, the model reproduces the pandemic process's fundamental behavior without introducing any macroscopic assumptions.

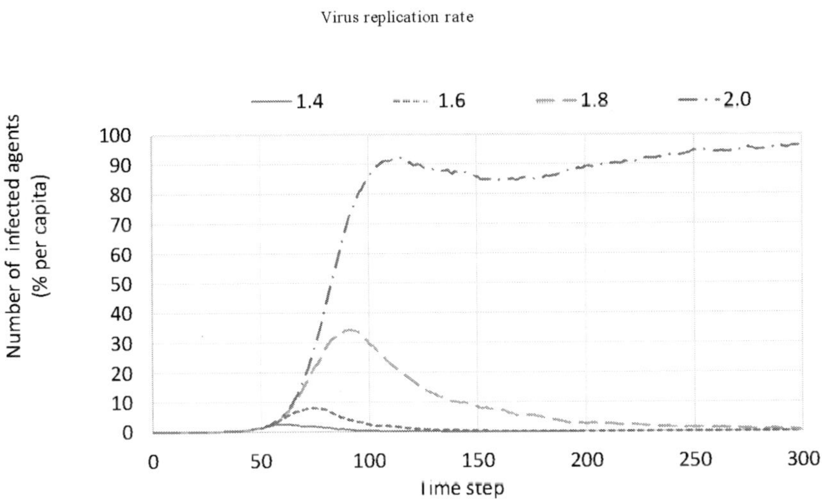

Figure 2. Effect of the virus replication rate on the number of infected agents.

We can also examine the numbers of newly infected and newly recovered agents. The number of newly infected agents, which was initially one, increases drastically, peaks, then decreases, a trend stemming from agent interactions as shown in Figure 3. A similar trend of increase and decrease appears in the number of recovered agents because of the effects of innate immune cells and antibodies, as shown in Figure 4.

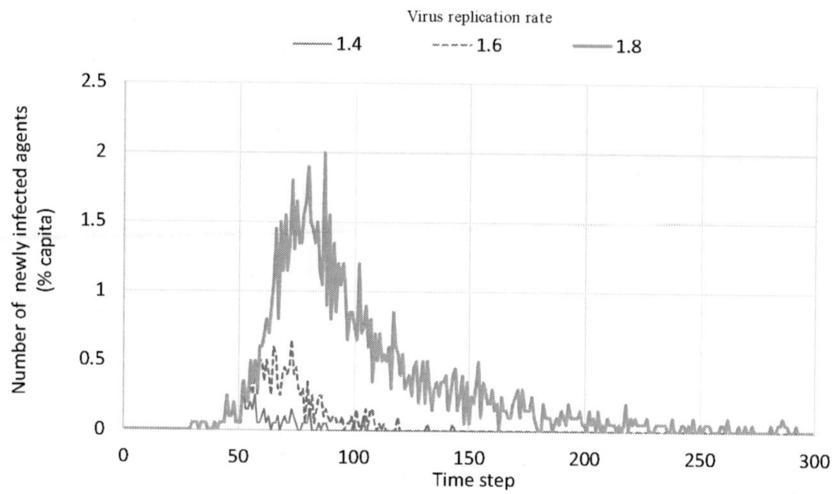

Figure 3. Effect of virus replication rate on the number of newly infected agents.

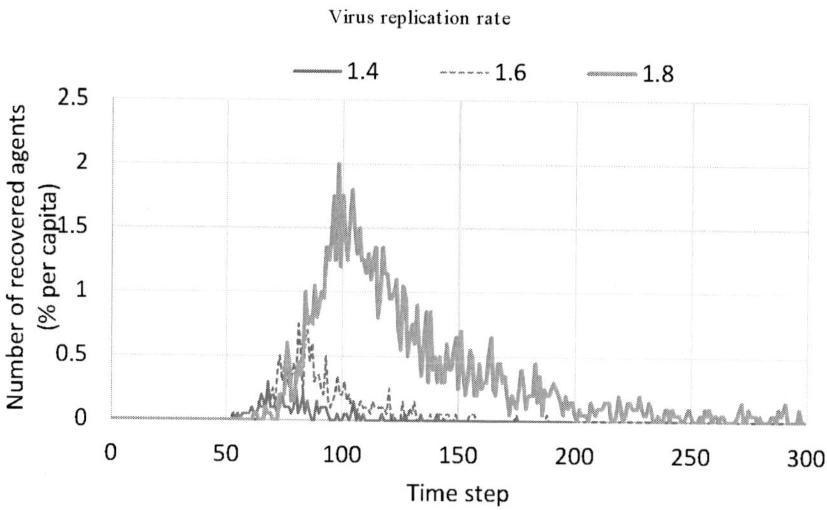

Figure 4. Effect of virus replication rate on the number of newly recovered agents.

The Relationship among Newly Infected, Newly Recovered and Total Infected Agents

Figure 5 shows the numbers of newly infected, newly recovered, and total infected agents as a function of time. Note that the total number of infected agents peaks at the period between the peaks for the numbers of newly infected and recovered agents. More precisely, the total number of infected agents reaches its maximum at the point where the number of newly infected agents equals the number of newly recovered agents as given in Figure 6. This is evident from the defined expression of the total number of infected agents, as shown in Equation (6). Namely, when the total number of infected agents peaks, its value in this period equals that of the previous period. Because the present model is assumed to neglect the death rate, this condition is satisfied when the number of newly infected agents equals the number of recovered agents, as seen in Equation (6).

$$N_{infected}^{t+1} = N_{infected}^{t} + N_{newly\ infected}^{t} - N_{newly\ recovered}^{t} - N_{newly\ dead}^{t}$$

$$\begin{aligned} where,\ & N_{infected} : Number\ of\ the\ infected \\ & N_{newly\ infected} : Number\ of\ the\ newly\ infected \\ & N_{Newly\ dead} : Number\ of\ the\ newly\ dead \\ & t : period \end{aligned} \tag{6}$$

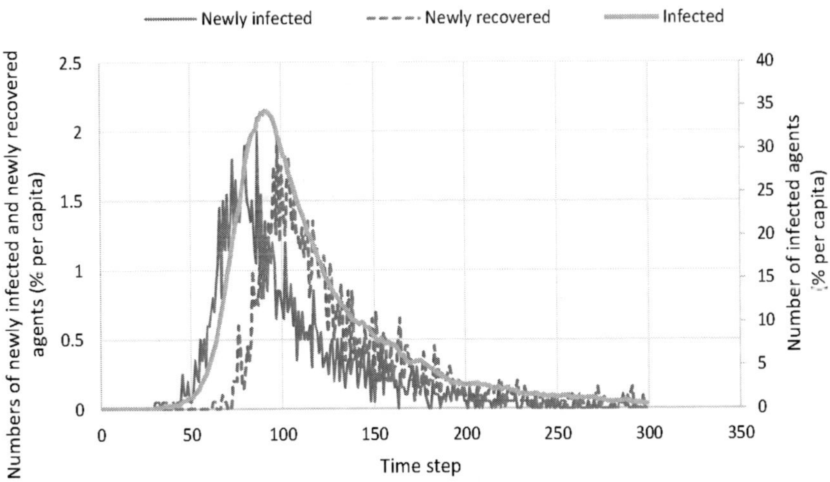

Figure 5. Changes in the numbers of newly infected, newly recovered and total infected agents (virus replication rate: 1.8).

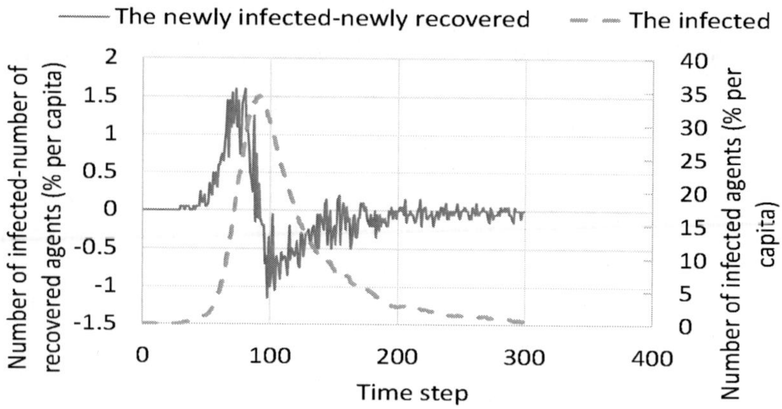

Figure 6. Change in the total number of infected agents and the difference between the numbers of newly infected and newly recovered agents (virus replication rate: 1.8).

Behavior of the Number of Viruses within Each Agent during Infection Spread and Convergence

This model can calculate the number of viruses within each agent at each time step. The aggregate variables, such as the numbers of infected agents and recovered agents, are evaluated based on this value at each time step, as explained in the previous section describing the model. Figure 7 shows an example of the change in each agent's number of viruses in the first stage of infection spread. In this example, the virus replication rate and the maximum traveling distance are assumed to be 1.8 and 100, respectively. Figure 7 shows how infections propagate from agent to agent in this artificial system. This example of calculated results shows that Agent 1 is the only infected agent initially, and Agent 13 is infected by Agent 1 at time step 4. The next agent who is infected by Agent 1 is Agent 155 at time step 25. However, before Agent 155 is infected, Agent 13 infects Agent 1373 at time step 6, and infection propagates from Agent 1373 to Agent 1019, and from Agent 1019 to Agent 1911. In this way, this model allows individual tracking of the details of the infection process. The same is true for the recovery process.

Note that, in Figure 7, the slope of the change in the number of viruses appears positive or negative just after the infection. Here, the slope in the number of viruses depends on the relative magnitude of the relationship between the virus replication rate and the immune attack rate. If the effect of replication is larger than that of immune cells, the slope becomes positive, and vice versa. Moreover, note that, after a certain infection period, the slopes of all agents become negative, and their magnitudes become greater due to the emergence of antibodies. The slope's magnitude is different for each agent due to the agent-specific value of the antibody attack rate. Thus, the number of viruses within each infected agent decreases with time, at least after antibody emergence.

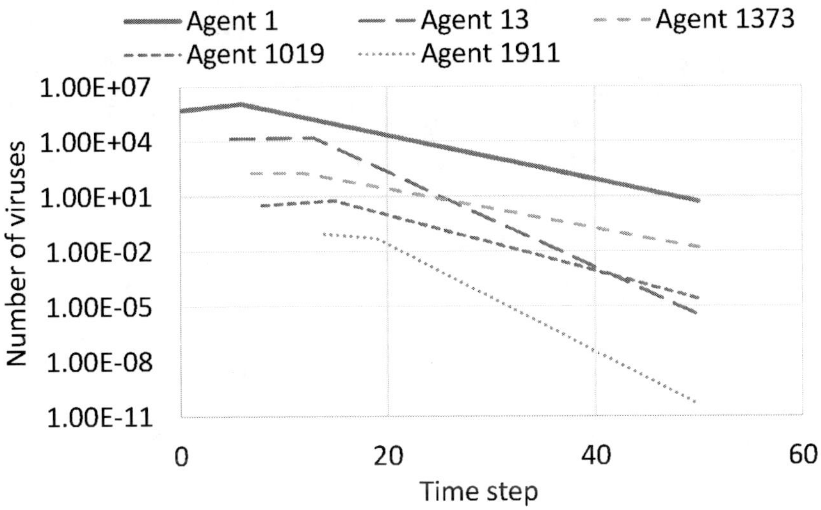

Figure 7. Changes in the number of viruses of agents who are sequentially infected during the initial stage of infection spread (infection spread sequence: Agent 1→13→1373→1019→1911, virus replication rate: 1.8).

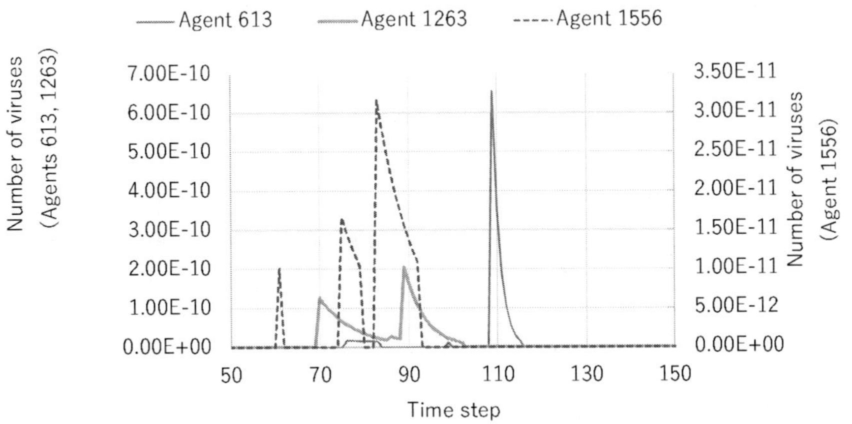

Figure 8. Examples of cases where agents are infected multiple times. The calculation conditions are the same as those in Figure 7.

During infection and recovery, an agent could be infected multiple times. Figure 8 shows such an example. Note that, as seen for Agent 1556 in Figure 3, the rate of propagation of viruses may change over time, as seen by a decrease in the number of viruses, due to the emergence of antibodies. In Agent 613, there is no change in rate during the decrease in the number of viruses, indicating that the agent has recovered before the emergence of antibodies. Whether antibodies emerge or not depends on the number of viruses at the time of infection, the agent-specific value of the antibody-emerging period, and the immune cells' virus attack rate.

Figures 9 and 10 show the trends in the number of viruses at the time of infection during infection spread and convergence. The number of viruses within each agent at the time of infection decreases during infection spread and convergence, as shown in Figure 9.

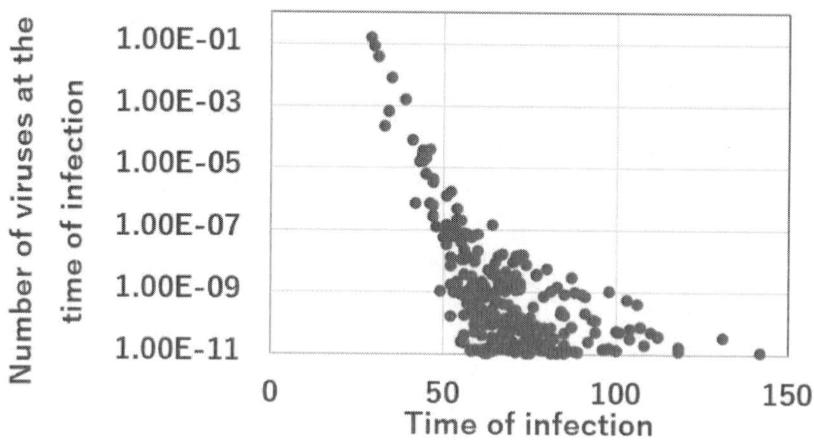

Figure 9. Number of viruses at the time of infection as a function of time during infection spread and convergence (virus replication rate: 1.6).

This trend reflects the effects of the virus-releasing rate, the virus-absorbing rate, the virus attack rate of immune cells or antibodies, and the virus replication rate. Namely, when an infection occurs, a healthy person receives a portion of the viral particles released by the infected person due to a cough or other means, and the emitted viral particles are a portion of the viruses possessed by the infected person, which decreases with time if the effect of the virus attack rate of immune cells or antibodies is larger than the effect of virus replication rate. Thus, the number of viruses at the time of infection decreases during the propagation process because viral particles transferred from an infected to a healthy person are only a portion of the viruses held by that infected person, which decreases with time due to the effect of immunity. It is also observed that total number of viruses in the system also decreases with time due to the effect of immunity.

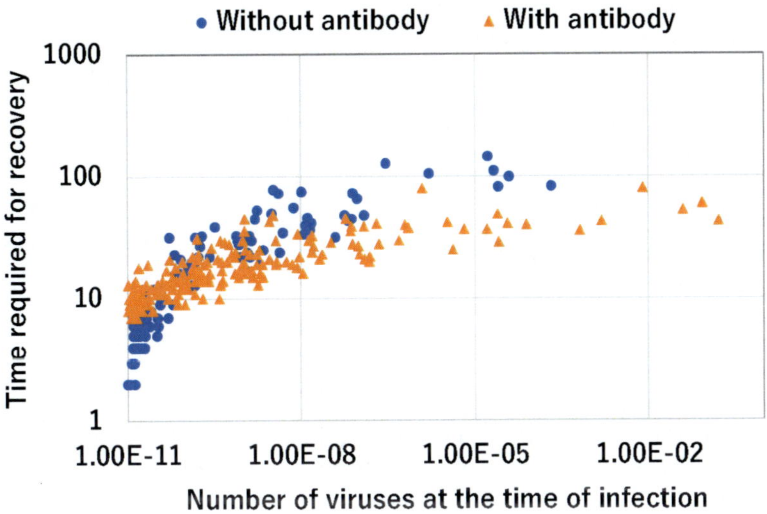

Figure 10. Time required for recovery as a function of the number of viruses at the time of infection (virus replication rate: 1.6).

Note that, as the number of viruses at the time of infection decreases, the time required for recovery becomes shorter, as shown in Figure 5. This indicates that the time necessary for an infected person to recover becomes shorter with time as the number of viruses at the time of infection decreases during the process of infection spread and convergence.

The Behavior of Infection Spread and Recovery When the Pandemic Does Not Converge

Let us examine how the infection spreads in the case where the pandemic does not converge from the viewpoint of the number of viruses. Figure 11 shows the changes with time in the numbers of newly infected, newly recovered, and infected agents when the virus replication rate is 2.0, under which conditions the pandemic does not converge, as already illustrated in Figure 2. Note that the number of newly infected agents initially increases and then decreases after reaching its maximum until the time step of around 100 and the number of newly recovered agents at one point exceeds the number of newly infected agents. This trend is one of the features in the case of pandemic convergence, as given in Figure 9. However, the number of newly infected agents increases again after the time step of around 100 and the number of newly recovered agents never exceeds the number of newly infected agents after the time step of 150, as shown in Figure 11.

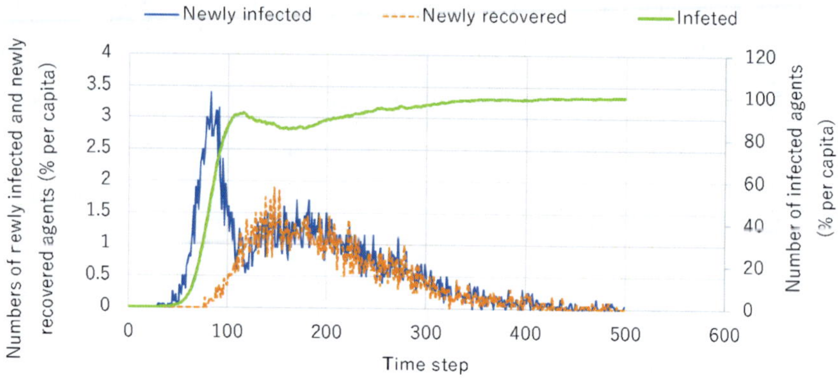

Figure 11. The changes in the numbers of newly infected, newly recovered, and total infected agents when virus replication rate is 2.0 where the pandemic does not converge (virus replication rate: 2.0).

Let us examine what is happening before and after the time step of around 100. Figure 12 shows the number of viruses possessed by each agent at the time of infection. Note that each agent's number of viruses at the time of infection initially decreases until the time step of around 100, but it increases again after that.

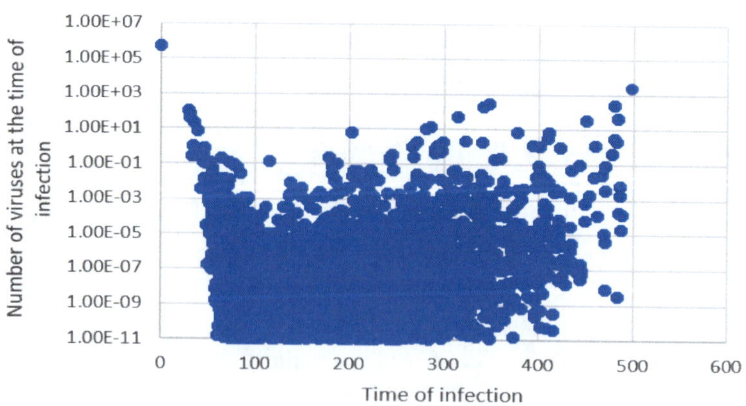

Figure 12. Number of viruses at the time of infection as a function of the time of infection (virus replication rate: 2.0).

These results indicate that if there is more than one person in the system whose effect of immunity is less than the effect of virus replication, the pandemic never converges. This is because the number of viruses of such agents continually increases unless they are entirely isolated. Meeting this individual increases the number of viruses of other agents at the time of infection, meaning that their recovery takes time. This causes the repeated infection of such agents during recovery. Thus, the number of viruses of such agents increases, and they never recover even if their immune response is large enough compared with the effect of virus replication.

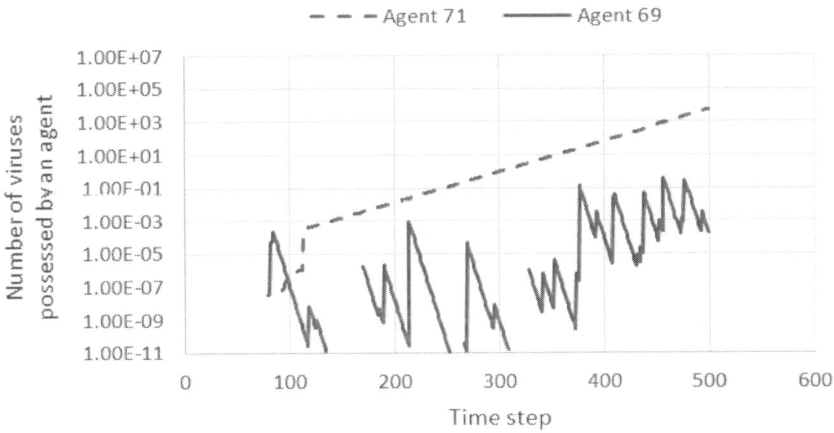

Figure 13. Examples of the change in the number of viruses of agents whose effect of immunity is smaller (agent 71) or larger (agent 69) than the effect of virus replication (virus replication rate: 2.0).

Figure 13 shows examples of the change in the number of viruses of agents whose effect of immunity is smaller (agent 71) or larger (agent 69) than the effect of virus replication. Close observation revealed the details of infection and recovery of each agent as follows.

Agent 71 in Figure 13 was first infected at time 92 and antibodies emerged at time 101. The number of viruses kept increasing even after the emergence of antibodies, showing that the effect of immunity could not overcome the effect of virus replication in the case of agent 71. The number of viruses of agent 71 drastically increased at time 113 because of reinfection due to meeting agent 46, who had a large number of viruses, and it subsequently kept increasing while repeatedly infecting others and being infected by others.

In contrast, agent 69 in Figure 13 was first infected at time 79 and the antibodies emerged at time 86. This agent's number of viruses decreased after antibody emergence, although it increased before then. This trend indicates that the effect of immunity in the case of agent 69 overcomes the effect of virus replication after the emergence of antibodies. Agent 69 recovered once at time 136 but was infected again at time 170. Since then, this agent's number of viruses repeatedly increased and decreased due the repeated cycles of infection and recovery. Note that, during the repeated infection and recovery, the number of viruses gradually increased with the passing of time. This trend is because the number of viruses of agent 69 at the time of infection increased during the repeated infections as the number of viruses of other agents who infected agent 69, such as agent 71, increased with the passing of time, causing an increase in the time required for recovery. Thus, agent 69 was repeatedly reinfected during recovery by others whose number of viruses continually increased. Agent 69 thus never recovers, even if this agent's immune response is sufficient to outcompete virus replication.

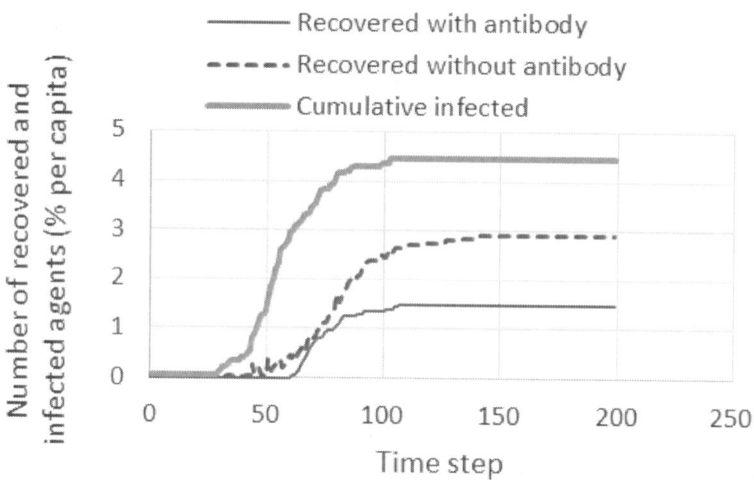

Figure 14. Changes in the numbers of recovered agents with and without antibodies and the cumulative number of infected agents (virus replication rate: 1.4).

The Ratio of Recovered Agents with Antibodies to the Total Number of Recovered Agents

Because the present model neglects the occurrence of death, all infected agents eventually recover in the case where the effect of immunity is larger than the effect of virus replication for all agents in the system. Whether the infected agents recover with antibodies depends on the virus replication rate and agent-specific virus attack rate. As shown in Figure 14, in the case of a low virus replication rate, such as 1.4, two-thirds of the infected agents recover without antibodies. In contrast, at a replication rate of 1.8, more than 90% of recovered agents possess antibodies, as shown in Figure 15. In any case, all infected people recover regardless of the emergence of antibodies. This indicates that, whether those who recover with antibodies constitute most of the population is not a crucial factor in determining whether the pandemic ends.

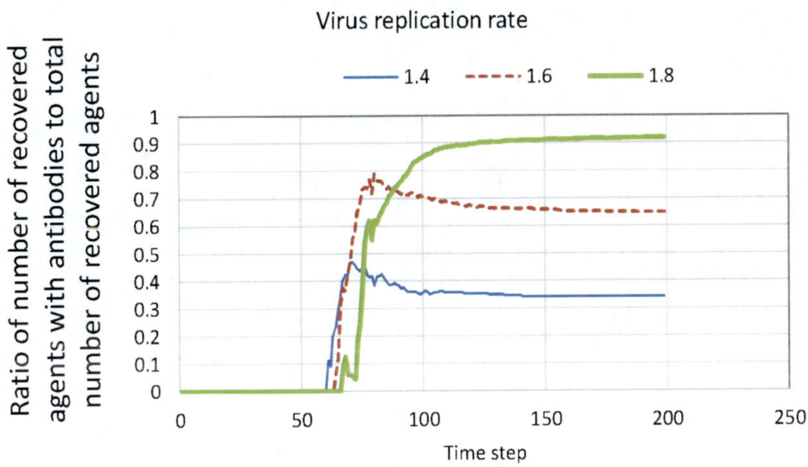

Figure 15. Effect of virus replication rate on the ratio of the number of recovered agents with antibodies to the total number of recovered agents.

Effect of the Virus Replication Rate on the Number of Infected Neighbors

In the present model, agents within a distance of 5 m are called neighbors. Neighbors who are infected are called infected neighbors.

Figure 16 demonstrates the effect of the virus replication rate on the average number of infected neighbors. Note that this pattern is very close to those of the infected and newly infected agents shown in Figures 2 and 3. There is a close relationship between the number of infected agents and the number of infected neighbors, as shown in Figure 17. The number of infected agents increases with the number of infected neighbors, as shown in Figure 18. The source of scattering in Figure 18 is considered to be the scattering of the number of viruses at the time of infection. These results indicate that the leading cause of infection spread is a healthy person encountering an infected person, the repetition of which increases the probability of other healthy persons meeting an infected person, causing a progressive increase in the number of infected agents.

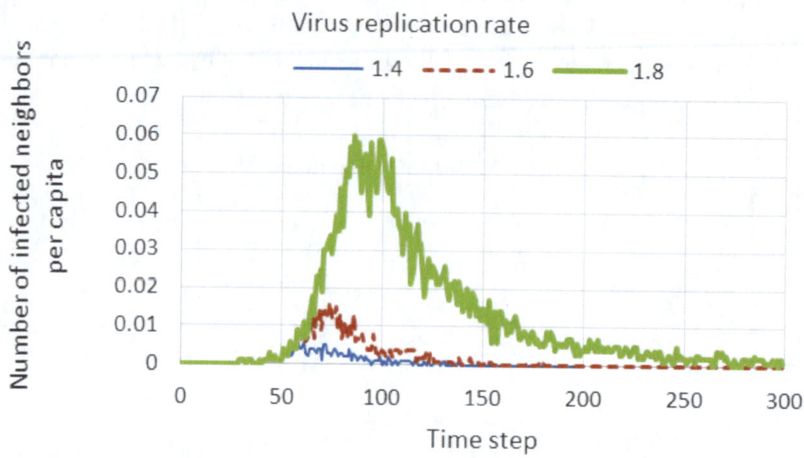

Figure 16. Effect of the virus replication rate on the average number of infected neighbors.

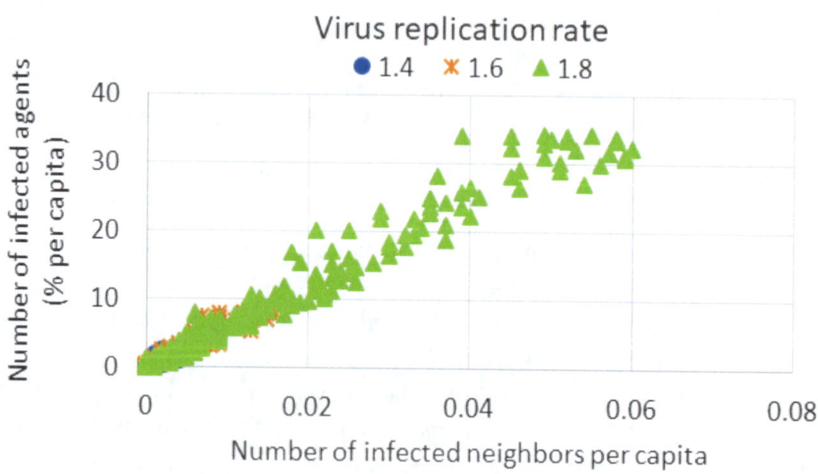

Figure 17. Relationship between the number of infected agents and the average number of infected neighbors.

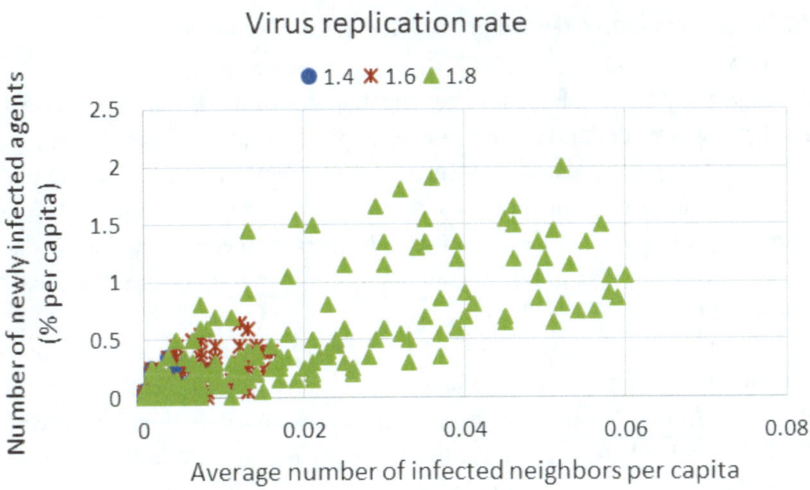

Figure 18. Relationship between the number of newly infected agents and the average number of infected neighbors.

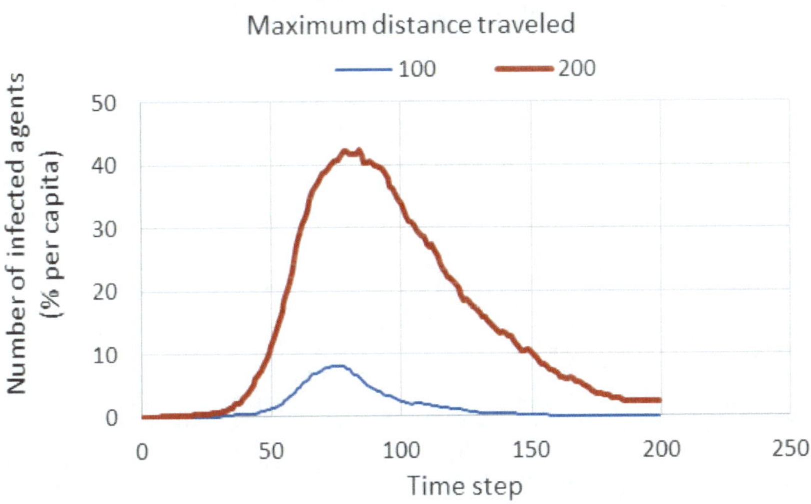

Figure 19. Effect of the maximum distance traveled on the total number of infected agents (virus replication rate: 1.6).

Effect of Maximum Distance Traveled on the Number of Infected Agents

Because the present model assumes that the movement is random in terms of its distance and direction, the probability of an uninfected agent meeting an infected agent depends on the maximum distance traveled. The calculated results presented in the previous sections correspond to cases where the maximum distance traveled is set as 100 m. How the estimated numbers of various groups are affected by doubling the maximum distance traveled can also be examined.

Figures 19 and 20 show the effect of the maximum distance traveled on the numbers of total infected and newly infected agents, respectively. Note that both factors became much more significant by doubling the maximum distance traveled. The reason for this tendency is that, as shown in Figure 21, as the maximum distance traveled increases, the average number of infected neighbors increases; that is, an uninfected agent can meet infected neighbors more often.

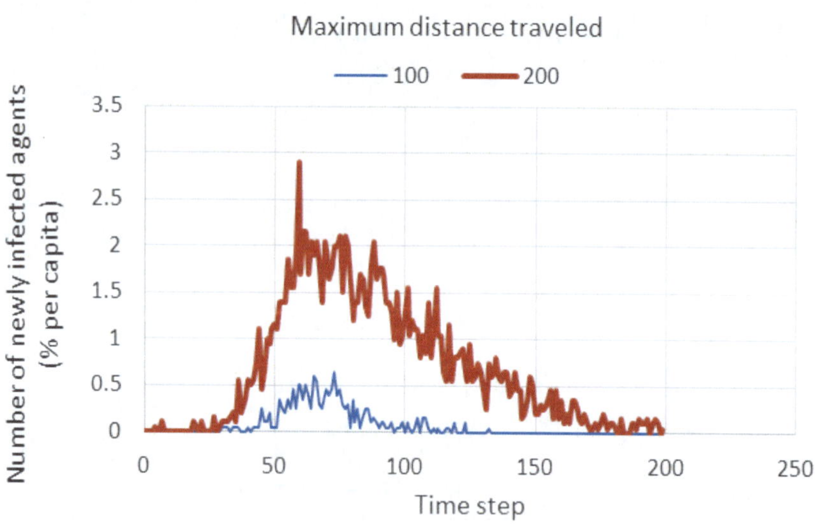

Figure 20. Effect of the maximum distance traveled on the number of newly infected agents (virus replication rate: 1.6).

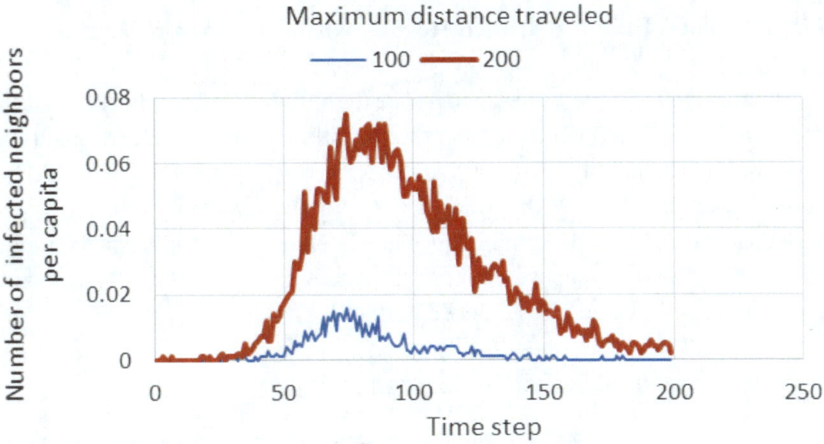

Figure 21. Effect of the maximum distance traveled on the average number of infected neighbors (virus replication rate: 1.6).

Effect of Virus-Absorbing Rate on the Number of Infected Agents

Figure 22 shows the effect of the virus-absorbing rate on the number of infected agents; the number of infected agents drastically decreases as the virus-absorbing rate decreases. Thus, wearing a mask or engaging in infection prevention measures may be effective for decreasing the number of viral particles at the time of infection.

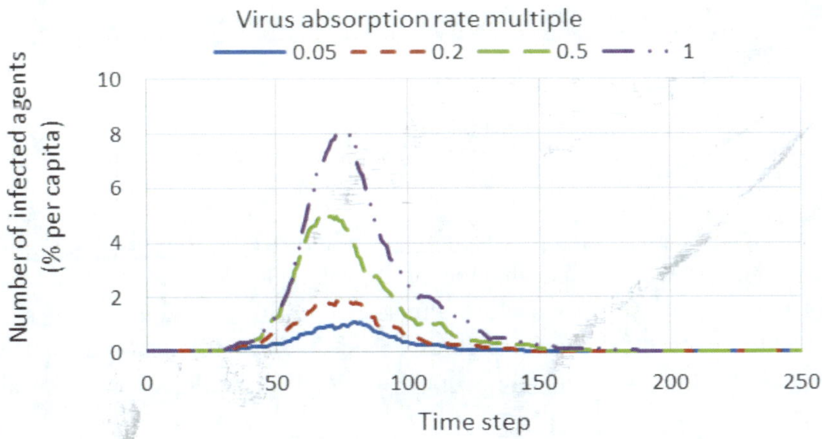

Figure 22. Effect of the virus-absorbing rate on the number of infected agents (virus replication rate: 1.6).

Comparison of the Calculated Results with Real-World Data

Figures 23 and 24 show the changes in the numbers of newly infected and recovered people and in the number of currently infected people, respectively, observed in Japan in 2020 for the SARS-CoV-2 pandemic (Worldmeter/coronavirus_updates, 2020). Note that the number of newly infected people peaked around April 15, the number of newly recovered people peaked around May 10, and both indices were almost the same around April 30. Additionally, the number of infected people peaked around April 30.

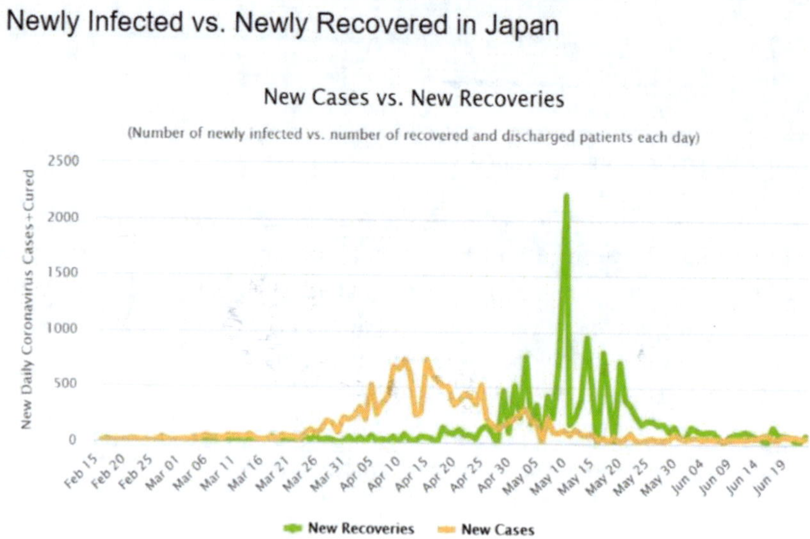

Figure 23. Changes in the numbers of newly infected and recovered people in Japan as of June 20, 2020.

Thus, the period at which the number of infected persons peaks coincides with the period at which the number of newly infected persons and the number of newly recovered persons are almost the same. This trend matches the calculated results shown in Figures 5 and 6. Thus, the model adequately reproduces the fundamental behavior of the numbers of infected and recovered persons.

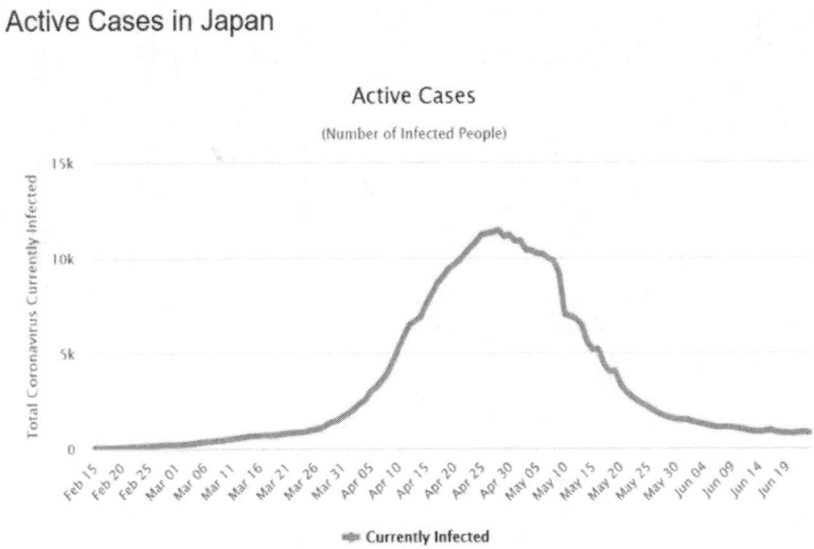

Figure 24. Change in the number of currently infected people in Japan as of June 20, 2020.

Implementing and Relaxing Restrictions on Movement and the Effect of the Virus-Absorbing Rate

In this section, the effects of various factors on the emergence of a re-increase in the number of infected persons, referred to here as a second wave, are analyzed. A re-increase in the number of infected persons after complete convergence of the pandemic, a real second wave, does not occur because the total number of viruses in the system becomes almost zero after convergence of the pandemic, as seen in Figure 9.

Effect of Implementing and Relaxing Restrictions on Movement

Figure 25 shows the changes in the number of infected agents under the base condition and the experimental conditions. In the experimental conditions, the maximum distance traveled is decreased to 0.2 times or 0.1 times, that is, to 20% or 10%, during the period between t=50 and t=100 and returns to the original value for the period after t=100. Notably, when the maximum traveling distance is decreased to 0.2 times, the number of newly infected agents initially decreases and then increases again after the end of the restriction; in other words, another wave of the pandemic arises. In contrast, when the maximum distance traveled is decreased to 0.1 times, that is, when the restrictions are applied strictly, only another weak wave of the pandemic occurs.

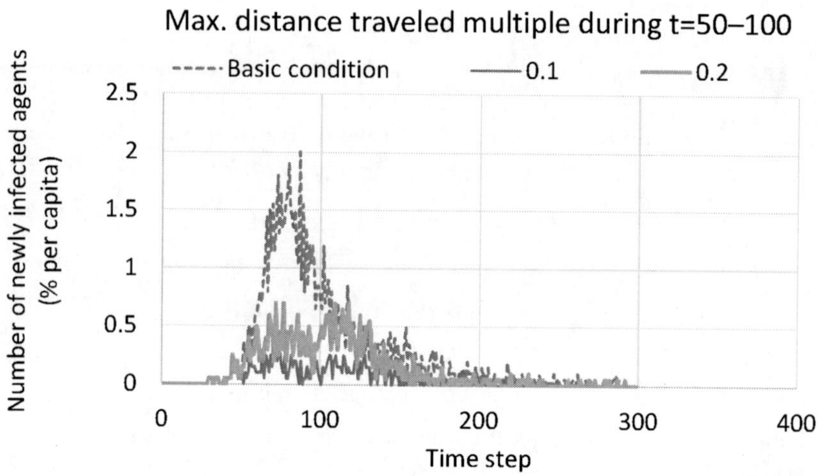

Figure 25. Effect of temporary restriction on distance traveled and its relaxation on the number of newly infected agents (virus replication rate: 1.8).

Similar behavior is observed in the average number of infected neighbors and the total number of infected agents, as shown in Figures 26 and 27, respectively. Namely, the emergence of another wave of the pandemic is remarkable in the case of loose restrictions, whereas it hardly occurs in the case of strict controls. The reason for this is that, in the case of strict controls, the number of infected agents just before relaxing the controls is small. Moreover, the number of viruses in infected individuals is also small, resulting in more rapid recovery, as suggested by Figures 9 and 10. Therefore, the probability of meeting an infected agent becomes low in the case of strict controls.

The number of recovered agents with antibodies is smaller in the case of strict controls on movement (Figure 28), indicating that the emergence of antibodies is not responsible for preventing a second wave of the pandemic because more people may recover without antibodies in the case of strict controls.

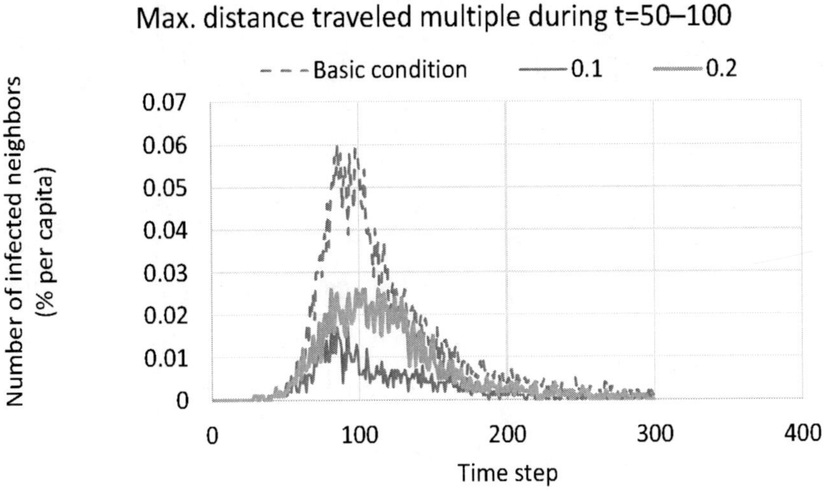

Figure 26. Effect of temporary restrictions of distance traveled and its relaxation on the number of infected neighbors (virus replication rate: 1.8).

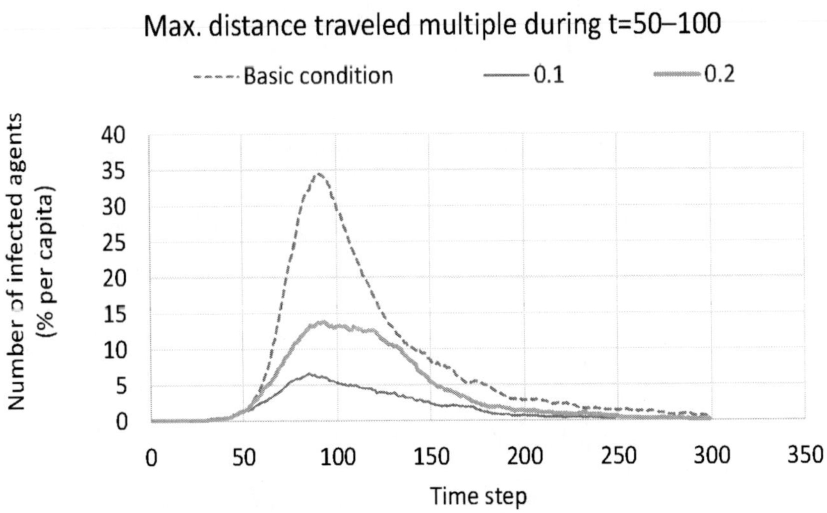

Figure 27. Effect of temporary restriction of distance traveled and its relaxation on the total number of infected agents (virus replication rate: 1.8).

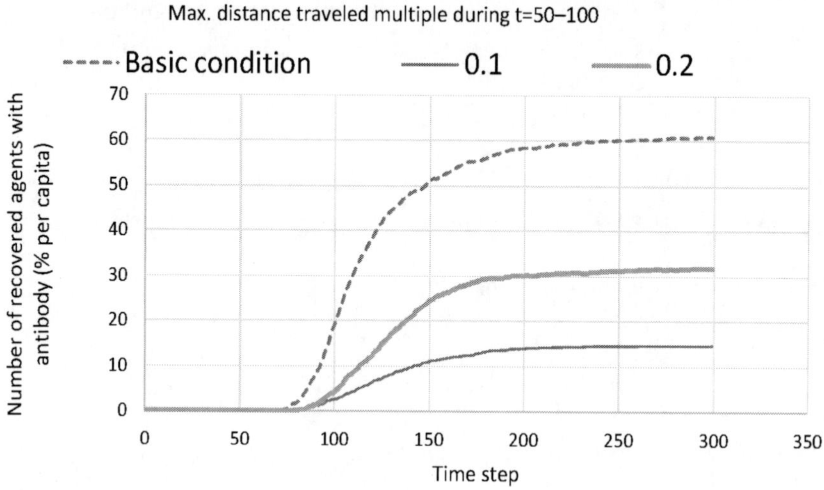

Figure 28. Effect of temporary restriction of distance traveled and its relaxation on the number of recovered agents with antibodies (virus replication rate: 1.8).

Effect of the Virus-Absorbing Rate on Infection Behavior during the Implementation and Relaxation of Restrictions on Movement

This section describes the effect of the virus-absorbing rate on infection behavior during the implementation and relaxation of restrictions on movement. Figure 29 shows the number of newly infected agents for different patterns of decrease of the virus-absorbing rate. Here, the maximum distance traveled is decreased to 0.2 times during only certain periods. There are three periods: t<50, t=50–100, and t>100. The virus-absorbing rate is set for each period, and the notations "1-1-1," "1-0.2-1," and "1-0.2-0.2" in Figure 29 represent a set of multiples for each period. For example, the notation "1-0.2-0.2" represents a pattern in which the virus-absorbing rate is decreased to 0.2 times in the second and third periods.

In the case of the 1-1-1 pattern, a second wave of the pandemic arises in the period after t=100 where regulation is released (Figure 29). In the case of the 1-0.2-1 pattern, the emergence of another wave of the pandemic is not remarkable, but the number of newly infected agents increases slightly in the period after t=100. In contrast, in the case of the 1-0.2-0.2 pattern, another wave of the pandemic does not arise, indicating that strict prevention measures against infection are quite effective for preventing the emergence of another wave of the pandemic. This tendency is more clearly observed in the total number of infected agents (Figure 30).

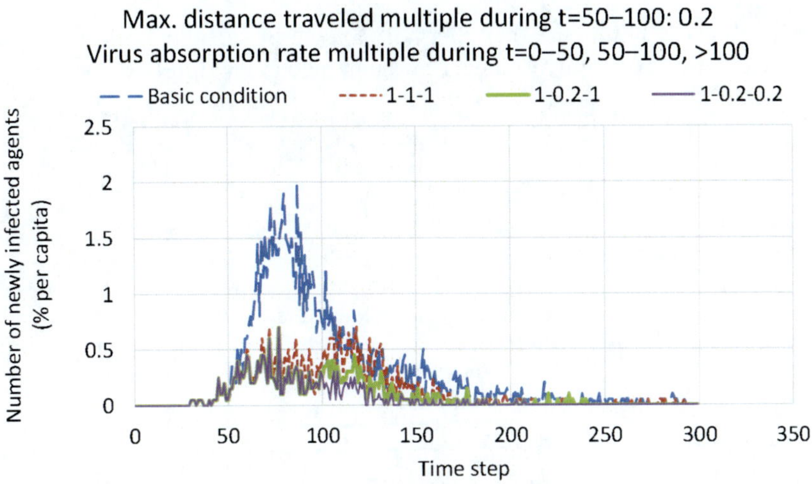

Figure 29. Effect of the virus-absorbing rate on the number of newly infected agents when movement restriction is applied (virus replication rate: 1.8).

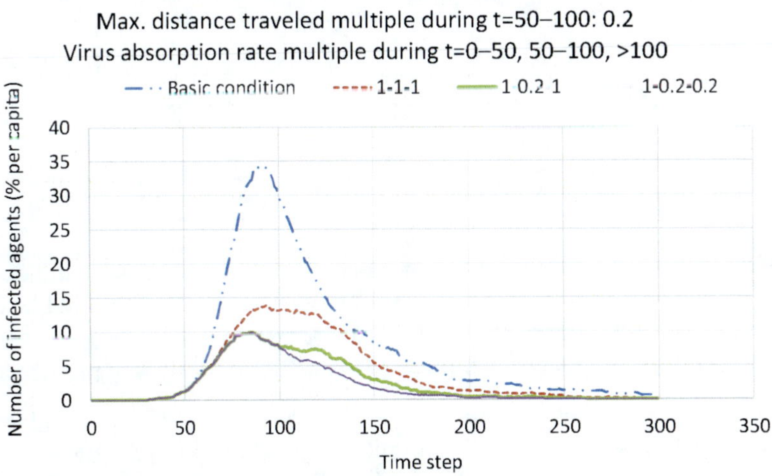

Figure 30. Effect of the virus-absorbing rate on the number of infected agents when movement restriction is applied (virus replication rate: 1.8).

A similar trend is also seen in the average number of infected neighbors (Figure 31). This indicates that the effect of the virus-absorbing rate on the number of newly infected agents is as follows. The decrease in the virus-absorbing rate decreases the number of viruses of infected individuals at the time of infection, which increases the number of newly recovered agents due to the increase in the recovery speed, as suggested by Figure 10. This in turn decreases the probability of a healthy agent meeting an infected agent.

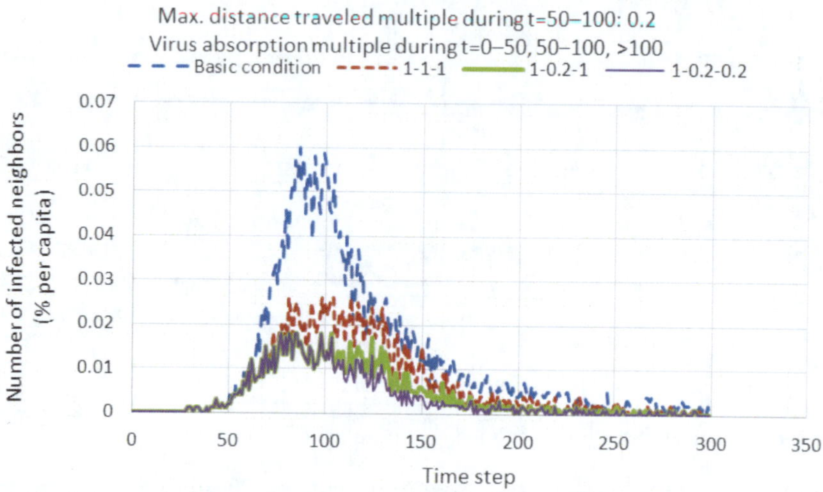

Figure 31. Effect of the virus-absorbing rate on the average number of infected neighbors when movement restriction is applied (virus replication rate: 1.8).

Infection Behavior When No Antibodies Are Present

Figure 32 shows the infection and recovery trends when no antibodies are present. Notably, the numbers of newly infected, newly recovered, and total infected agents exhibit patterns similar to those shown in Figure 5, which represents the case with antibodies. This indicates that the existence of antibodies is not an essential factor in the mechanism of the fundamental behavior of increasing and decreasing the number of infected agents.

However, in the case when no antibodies are present, the virus replication rate that is necessary for pandemic convergence is 1.3 in Figure 32, which is significantly lower than that in the case with antibodies, which is 1.8 as shown in Figure 5. If the virus replication rate is 1.4, the number of newly recovered agents never exceeds the number of newly infected agents and therefore the pandemic never converges, as shown in Figure 33. These results indicate that antibodies play a significant role in expanding the upper limit of the virus replication rate below which pandemic convergence can occur, although antibodies are not essential for the fundamental mechanism of infection and recovery.

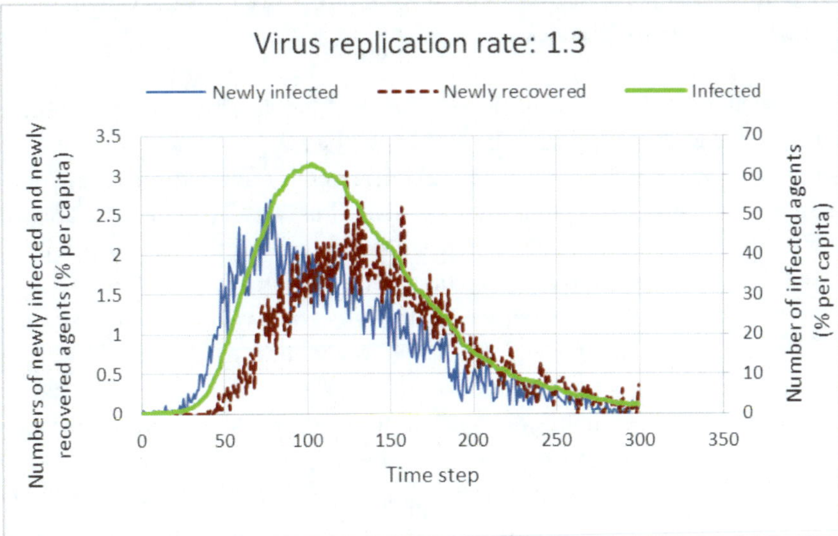

Figure 32. An example of the calculated numbers of newly infected, newly recovered, and total infected agents in the case without antibodies when the pandemic converges (virus replication rate: 1.3).

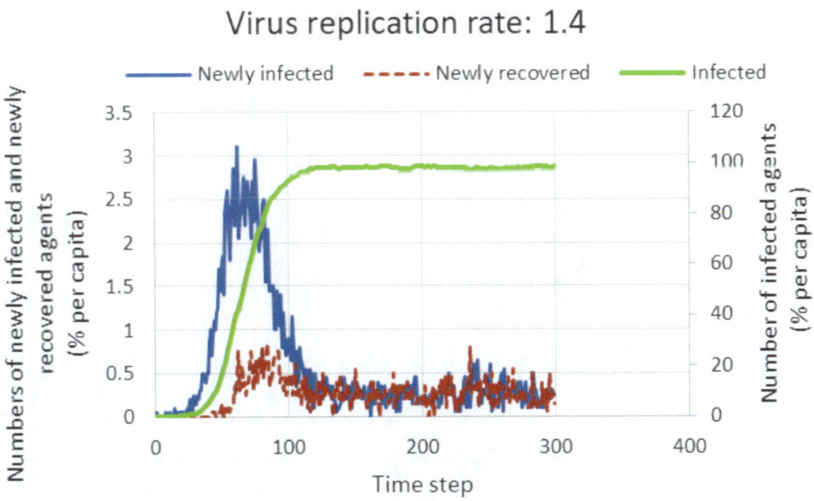

Figure 33. An example of the calculated numbers of newly infected, newly recovered, and total infected agents in the case without antibodies when the pandemic does not converge (virus replication rate: 1.4).

Infection Behavior When the Decreasing Increment of the Number of Viruses due to the Effect of Immune Cells or Antibodies Is Assumed to Be a Constant Value Independent of the Number of Viruses

The calculation described so far assumes that the decrease in the number of viruses due to immunity per time step is proportional to the number of viruses in that period, as given in Equation (2). Here, let us refer to the decrease in the number of viruses per time step as the virus attack count. A series of experiments was additionally conducted, assuming that the virus attack count is a constant value independent of the number of viruses in each period. This assumption corresponds to neglecting the effect of fever. The constant values and virus replication rates were varied widely in these experiments.

Figure 34 shows the influence of the virus replication rate on the number of infected agents under these conditions. Here, the constant value for the virus attack count is assumed to be 3 for immune cells and 5 for antibodies. These values correspond to ten times the virus attack rate for immune cells and antibodies, respectively. The virus replication rate is changed between 1.0 and 1.2. As shown in Figure 34, the pandemic converges when the virus replication rate is 1.05 or lower, and the pandemic does not converge when the virus replication rate is 1.1 or higher.

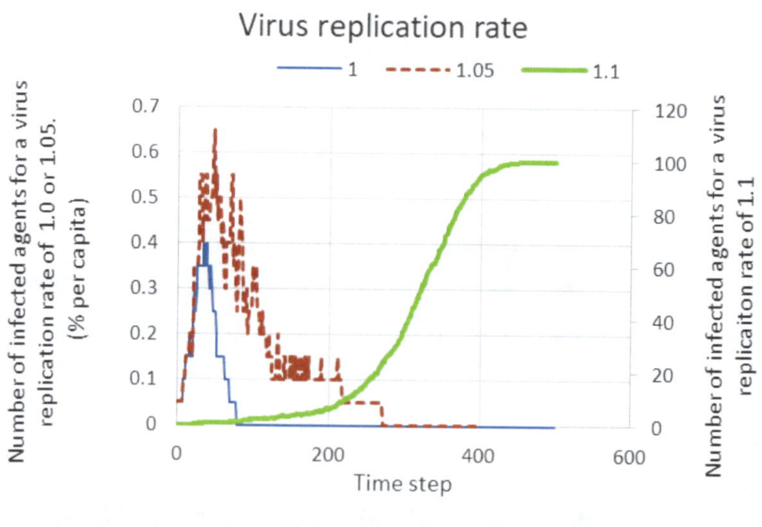

Figure 34. Influence of the virus replication rate on the number of infected agents when neglecting the effect of fever.

Interestingly, the trend of infection and recovery abruptly changes between the cases where the virus replication rate is 1.05 or lower or 1.1 or higher, despite the difference between them being very small. Namely, when the virus replication rate is 1.05, the maximum proportion of infected agents is 0.65% of the total population, while this value increases to around 100% when the virus replication rate is 1.1, as evident in Figure 34. This result indicates that if the virus attack count is assumed to be a constant value, namely if the effect of fever is neglected, the pandemic substantially does not occur, or the pandemic occurs and does not converge, where the critical virus replication rate is 1.1. In other words, under this assumption, the model cannot reproduce the actual pandemic phenomenon where the number of infected agents once drastically increases and then decreases. Thus, the most indispensable factor for reproducing the real pandemic phenomenon is the effect of fever, followed by the effect of antibodies which increases the upper limit of the virus replication rate for pandemic convergence.

Looking at the change over time in the number of viruses at the time of infection, it decreases as the time of infection increases when the pandemic converges although it is minor, as shown in Figure 35. This indicates that the total number of viruses in the system consistently decreases, thanks to the effect of immunity, so the pandemic converges.

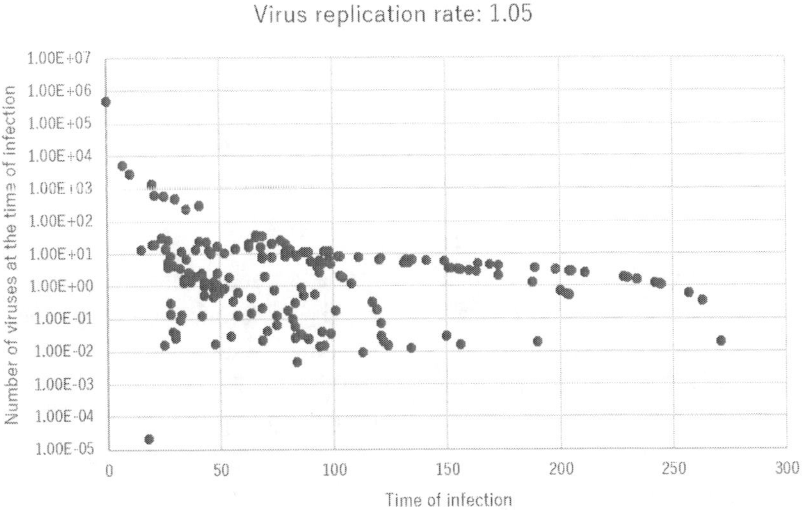

Figure 35. Number of viruses at the time of infection as a function of the time of infection, when the pandemic converges, showing that the total number of viruses in the system decreases due to the effect of immunity.

In contrast, when the virus replication rate is 1.1 (i.e., when the pandemic does not converge), the number of viruses at the time of infection increases from the very beginning of the pandemic, as shown in Figure 36. Besides, the number of newly recovered agents never exceeds the number of infected agents, as seen in Figure 37. As is evident by comparing these features with those shown in Figure 11 and Figure 12, these results indicate that when the virus replication rate is 1.1, many agents, in whom elimination of the virus by the immune system cannot keep up with virus replication, appear in the initial stage of the pandemic.

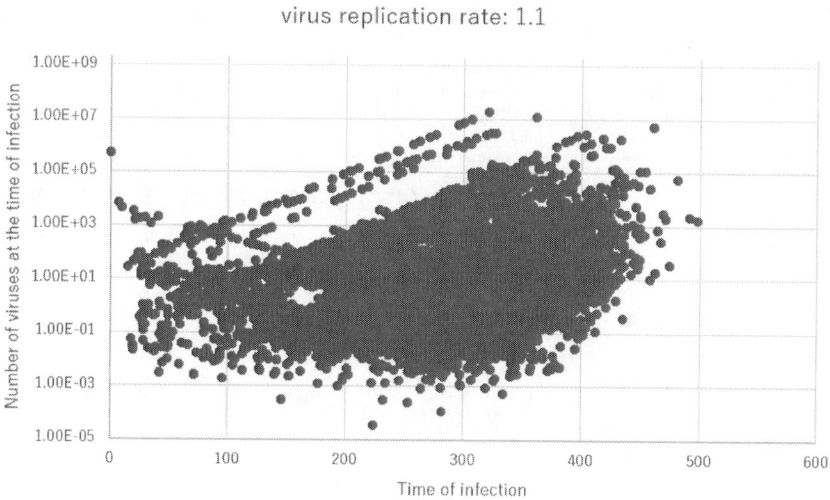

Figure 36. Number of viruses at the time of infection as a function of the time of infection, when the pandemic does not converge, showing that the total number of viruses in the system increases.

Similar results were also obtained in the additional experiments where the constant virus attack counts were assumed to be 100 times and 1000 times the virus attack rate for immune cells and antibodies. When increasing the attack count, the upper limit of the value of virus replication rate below which the pandemic converges slightly increases from 1.05 to 1.15.

Note that the critical value of the virus replication rate is 2.0 when the virus attack count is assumed to be proportional to the number of viruses and antibodies are present, as shown in Figure 2. This value decreases to 1.3 when antibodies are not present, as shown in Figure 32. As described above, when the virus attack count is assumed constant (i.e., when neglecting the effect of fever but assuming the effect of antibodies is present), this critical virus replication rate is between 1.05 and 1.15 for a wide range of virus attack counts. Here, we refer to these three cases as case 1, case 2, and case 3, respectively.

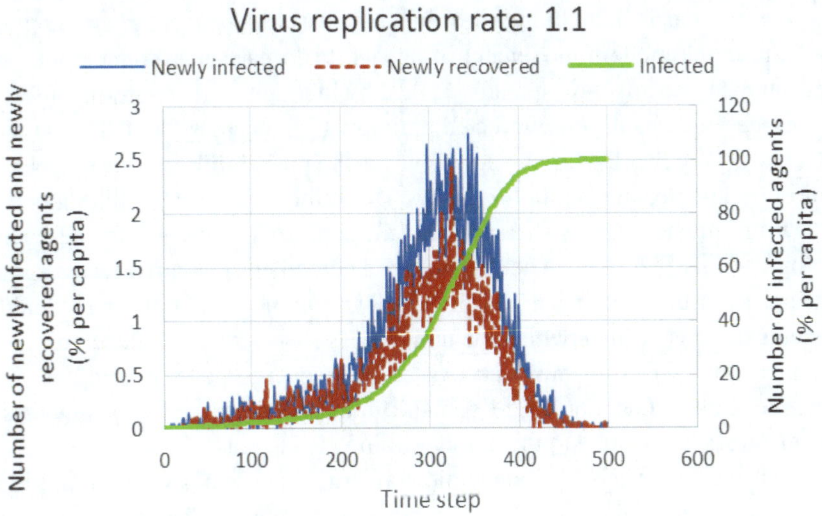

Figure 37. Calculated numbers of newly infected, newly recovered, and total infected agents, when the pandemic does not converge, showing that the number of newly recovered agents never exceeds the number of infected agents.

Also note that, below this critical rate of virus replication, the peak values of the number of infected agents gradually decreases as the virus replication rate decreases in case 1, as shown in Figure 2. This change becomes quite abrupt in case 3.

From these results, it is concluded that the most essential factor for pandemic convergence is that the rate of virus elimination by the immune system increases with an increase in the number of viruses in the human body. This factor corresponds to the fever associated with infection which increases the immunity. The next factor is the emergence of antibodies, whose effect on the rate of virus elimination is greater than that of innate immune cells. Both factors increase the upper limit of virus replication rate below which the pandemic converges.

Discussion

Fundamental Mechanisms of Infection Spread and Convergence

The present model analyzed the pandemic spread and convergence in the case where no particular countermeasures against the pandemic are applied, assuming the random movement of agents. If no particular countermeasures are applied, the infection spreads via healthy individuals encountering infected individuals if one or more infected individuals enter the system. The number of newly infected agents is dependent on the probability of a healthy agent meeting infected agents. In the early stage of the pandemic, the likelihood of meeting infected agents increases, so the number of newly infected agents progressively increases. After that stage, the number of newly infected agents decreases after reaching a peak because the number of uninfected healthy agents decreases. Meanwhile, the number of recovered agents depends on the number of infected agents who existed at a specific previous time because recovery takes time. For this reason, the number of recovered agents increases with a time lag relative to the number of infected agents.

In the case where the pandemic converges, the trends of the number of infected agents and the number of recovered agents are characterized by the number of newly infected agents becoming equal to the number of newly infected agents at a particular time, which is when the number of infected agents' peaks. The number of newly recovered agents exceeds the number of newly infected agents after that point.

Meanwhile, when the pandemic does not converge, the number of newly recovered agents never exceeds the number of newly infected agents. This is because the total number of viruses decreases with time in the former case and increases in the latter case. The consequence of this is evident from the calculated results of the behavior of the number of viruses shown in Figures 9, 12, 35, and 36. Figures 9 and 35 show the number of viruses at the time of infection in the case of pandemic convergence, which decreases with time. In contrast, Figure 36 shows that, when the pandemic does not converge, the number of viruses at the time of infection increases from the very beginning of the pandemic. Finally, Figure 12 shows the case in the middle, where the number of viruses at the time of being infected decreases and then increases.

These results indicate that the essential factor that characterizes pandemic convergence is the decreasing or increasing tendency of the number of viruses in the system during the pandemic. Close observation of the calculated results on the infection spread and recovery in terms of the number of viruses, as presented in Figure 13, revealed the reason why this factor is critical to whether or not the pandemic converges.

The agents in the system are heterogeneous in terms of the strength of their immune system. For a type of virus characterized by a particular rate of replication, there could be agents whose immune response cannot keep up with the speed of virus replication even after the emergence of antibodies, although many agents' immune responses can. If such agents with weak immunity are infected, the number of viruses would continually increase in their body because of virus replication.

The reason why the number of viruses at the time of infection starts to increase after showing a tendency to decrease at a particular time, as shown in Figure 12, is that such agents whose immune response cannot keep up with the virus replication rate are first infected at that time. In such cases, if such agents infect any other agents after that, the infected agents would receive a massive number of viruses at the time of infection. Therefore, recovery takes time, allowing repeated infections during the recovery period, as illustrated in Figure 13 as an example. Furthermore, during repeated infections, the number of viruses increases in the body, ending up in a state in which the immune response cannot keep up with the virus replication rate. Thus, such agents never recover, even if their innate immune response is adequate.

Thus, the critical factor that determines whether the pandemic converges or not is whether the system contains such agents whose immune response cannot keep up with the replication rate of the virus even if such agents are infected only once. If such agents exist in the system, moving around freely, the pandemic would never converge. Repeated infection also generates such agents. In contrast, if such agents do not exist in the system, pandemic converges even if the number of infected agents increases temporarily.

Another critical point for pandemic convergence is that the immunity of an agent increases upon the establishment of fever and the emergence of antibodies, which increases the upper limit of the virus replication rate below which the pandemic converges. According to the literature (Shu, T., 2020), the potency of immunity increases five-fold in response to a 1°C increase in body temperature. It is also well known (Eden, D., 2020) that innate immune cells are the first to attack viruses and, if necessary, antibodies emerge after a specific time to join the fight against the viruses. Thus, if an individual is infected, resulting in an increase in the number of viruses in the body, the body temperature will rise, which increases the potency of immunity due to innate immune cells. In many cases, people recover due to this effect of innate immune cells. However, for people with repeated infection or weak immunity, this effect of innate immune cells is insufficient to keep up with the virus replication, and antibodies emerge to join the fight against the viruses. Therefore, we can understand that humans have a mechanism for increasing immunity by increasing their body temperature and producing antibodies when the number of viruses in the body becomes large, compared with the effect of immunity due to infection and virus replication.

In the present study, the role of fever is modeled in that the immune response increases with an increasing number of viruses, as presented in Equation (2). The role of antibodies is modeled in that antibodies emerge when the immunity is insufficient to keep up with virus replication, having a more significant rate of virus attack, as presented in Equation (2) and Equation (3).

Note that the acceptable upper limit of the virus replication rate for the present study's pandemic convergence increases upon adding the roles of fever and antibodies. Namely, it was 1.05, 1.3, and 1.8 in the cases without the role of fever with antibodies, upon incorporating the role of fever without antibodies, and upon containing both roles, respectively, as explained in section 4.4.

From these results, we can conclude that the conditions that characterize pandemic convergence are as follows.

1. Fever and antibodies, which increase immunity, play indispensable roles for pandemic convergence for a wide range of virus replication rates. Among these factors, the role of fever is the most essential. Luckily, both of these roles are incorporated in every human being, because of which humans have survived for eons, overcoming every kind of pandemic.
2. Agents whose immunity cannot keep up with the rate of virus replication should not be included in the system for pandemic convergence. Such agents could arise in the system if any individuals are repeatedly infected in a short period.
3. In the body of such agents, the virus replicates indefinitely, thus increasing the number of viruses received by other agents when they infect them, thereby ensuring that the pandemic never converges. In general, such agents having many viruses may develop severe disease and are more likely to be isolated in hospital or elsewhere. Therefore, such agents need to be detected and isolated from the system quickly for pandemic convergence.

In summary, the fundamental mechanism of infection spread is the progressive increase in the probability of a healthy person meeting an infected person. The mechanism of convergence is that this probability decreases during the infection process due to the increased number of recovered people. Moreover, the rise of body temperature and the emergence of antibodies play essential roles in recovery from infection and the convergence of the pandemic because they increase the upper limit of virus replication for pandemic convergence.

Notably, once the pandemic ultimately converges in a system, an additional pandemic, namely, a second wave, never occurs unless infected people outside the system newly enter it. This is because the total number of viruses in a closed system decreases during the pandemic due to the effect of immunity. Moreover, under the condition that the pandemic finally converges, the person who becomes ill seriously with a very high body temperature is the person who is infected repeatedly without notifying infection, taking a large number of viruses in a short period before reaching recovery. Therefore, identifying and isolating only infected individuals is essential for pandemic convergence. This should be applied at national borders, airports, and densely populated places, such as commercial establishments and public transport.

A Proposed Strategy for Controlling the Pandemic While Protecting the Economy

Restricting the movement of people is an effective measure to control the spread of infection. However, movement restrictions cause economic activity to stagnate, thus weakening the economy. Therefore, to prevent infection spread while minimizing the impact on the economy, it is essential to reduce the probability that healthy people, who are the majority, encounter infected people, who are the minority.

In this context, the most fundamental strategy to control the spread of infection while minimizing the impact on the economy is to identify infected individuals and isolate them from healthy people. It is not necessary to control the movement of all people. Identifying infected people can be achieved by monitoring body temperature and performing PCR tests. Thus, the following measures are proposed as effective ways to prevent an impact on the economy and control infection spread. We can control the pandemic without harming the economy by employing these countermeasures.

1. Identifying severely infected individuals and isolating them or restricting their movement as much as possible. Severely infected people are those with a fever, which might exceed 38°C or at least 37.5°C. PCR tests can only identify whether a person is negative or positive, but they cannot determine the severity of infection. Moreover, false negative PCR test results are possible. In contrast, body temperature is a sign of being infected that also provides information about the severity of the disease. A higher body temperature generally indicates that the person is more severely infected. Therefore, measuring body temperature is the most reasonable and convenient way to identify infected individuals. This measure is essential at national borders, such as airports, to prevent infected individuals from entering a country.
2. Refusing entry of those suspected of being severely infected at national borders, such as at airports, as well as in densely populated places, such as commercial establishments. Body temperature measurement is the most reasonable and convenient way to identify such people. The critical temperature for refusing entry could be around 37.5°C. Irrespective of the absolute value, this measure would reduce the probability of healthy people encountering infected ones, thereby effectively controlling the spread of infection.
3. Establishing preventive measures in densely populated places, such as introducing ventilation, in addition to measuring body temperature at the entrances. Infection could occur via physical contact, droplets, or the airborne route. The difference between droplets and airborne infection is reported to relate to droplet size, with a threshold of 5 μm, according to the literature. Therefore, in the case of airborne infection, the viral particles could be released from an infected person and transferred to healthy people every time they breathe during a stay in an enclosed space. In such cases, people could be infected multiple times, causing repeated increases in the number of viruses in the body. Therefore, ventilation in such densely populated places might be essential to prevent the spread of infection.
4. Identifying infection by self-monitoring body temperature and then isolating oneself. If many infected individuals regulate their own behavior after monitoring their body temperature, this may significantly reduce the likelihood of a healthy person encountering an infected one, thus reducing the number of new infections.

5. Wearing a mask in densely populated places. This reduces virus emission from infected individuals and virus absorption by healthy individuals, which is modeled in the present study by introducing a virus-releasing rate and virus-absorbing rate. Note that the necessity of this measure depends on the individuals and the location.

Conclusion

An agent-based infection model that incorporates the roles of immune cells, antibodies, and viral particles was constructed in this study. Using this model, the effects of various factors on the spread and convergence of infection were analyzed, and the calculated results were compared with real-world data. The obtained results can be summarized as follows:

1. The present model well reproduced the qualitative features of the chronological patterns in the numbers of newly infected, newly recovered, and total infected agents observed in the real world.
2. The factors of the model indispensable for reproducing phenomena of the actual pandemic are the roles of fever and antibodies, where the former is modeled as the effect of immunity increasing with an increasing number of viruses and the latter is modeled as antibodies emerging when immunity is insufficient to keep up with virus replication, given that antibodies are associated with a more significant rate of virus attack.
3. The fundamental mechanism for the spread of infection is a progressive increase in the probability of a healthy person encountering an infected person, while the primary mechanism for convergence of the pandemic is a progressive decrease in the above probability as the number of recovered individuals increases.
4. The critical factor that determines whether the pandemic converges or not is whether in the system there are agents whose immune response cannot keep up with the virus replication rate. If such agents exist in the system, moving around freely, the pandemic will never converge. Repeated infection also generates such agents. In contrast, without such agents, the pandemic converges even if the number of infected agents increases temporarily.
5. The upper limit of the rate of virus replication for pandemic convergence increases when the effects of fever and the emergence

of antibodies are introduced into the model. The effect of fever is modeled as the potency of immunity increasing with an increase in the number of viruses, which is the most essential factor for the pandemic convergence.

6. Under the condition that the pandemic finally converges, the person who becomes ill seriously with a very high body temperature is the person who is infected repeatedly without notifying infection, taking a large number of viruses in a short period before reaching recovery.
7. This model also reproduced the re-increase in the number of infected individuals (i.e., another wave) after relaxing the temporary restriction on people's movement. However, once the pandemic ultimately converges, a second wave would never occur unless severely infected people from outside newly enter the system.
8. To control the spread of infection while minimizing the impact on the economy, it is essential to identify infected individuals, especially severely infected ones, and restrict the behavior of these infected individuals only. Measuring body temperature is an effective way of identifying such people, The identification and isolation of infected individuals are particularly essential at national borders, such as at airports, as well as at the entrances to densely populated places such as commercial establishments and public transport.
9. Self-monitoring of one's body temperature and restricting one's movement, if necessary, is also considered adequate for pandemic convergence. With this measure, a person can avoid repeated infection before reaching recovery and, therefore, will never become ill seriously. It is considered that the pandemic might quickly converge if most individuals do this measure.

References

Anderson R. M. and May, R. M. (1991) *Infectious Diseases of Humans: Dynamics and Control,* Oxford University Press, New York.

Bailey N. T. J. (1975) *The Mathematical Theory of Infectious Diseases* (Mathematics in Medicine series) Graffin, London.

Britton T. and Ball F. (2019) *Stochastic Epidemic Models with Inference* (Lecture Notes in Mathematics), Springer.

Eden David, (2020) *"Beyond the antibodies: How our immune system may protect us against COVID-19 infection,"* Accessed August 18. https://abcnews.go.com/Health/antivodies-/story?id=71879020.

Epstein J. M. and Axtell R. (1995) *Growing Artificial Societies, (Social Science from the Bottom Up),* MIT Press, London.

Li M. Y. (2019) *An Introduction to Mathematical Modeling of Infectious Diseases (Mathematics of Planet Earth),* Springer.

Li Yan, Lawley A. Mark., Siscovick S. David, Zhang D., Pagan A. Jose (2016) Agent-Based Modeling of Chronic Diseases: A Narrative Reviews and _Future Research Directions, *Prev Chronic Dis.* May.26;13:E69. Doi:10.5888/pcd 13.150561.

Marchuk G. I. (2019) *Mathematical Modeling of Immune Response in Infectious Diseases (Mathematics and Its Applications),* Kluwer Academic Publishers.

Ogibayashi S. and Shinagawa K. (2020) Model Structure of Agent-Based Artificial System for Reproducing the Emergence of Bullying Phenomenon, In: *Proceedings of the 2018 Conference of the Computational Social Science Society of the Americas,* Springer, pp229-250.

Ogibayashi S. and Takashima K. (2017) Influence of Inefficiency in Government Expenditure on the Multiplier of Public Investment, *Comput Econ* 50:549-577, doi: 10.1007/210614-017-9671-y.

Ogibayashi S. and Takashima K. (2019) System Structure of Agent-Based Model Responsible for Reproducing Business Cycles and the Effect of Tax Reduction on GDP," In: *Journal on Policy and Complex Systems,* Vol.5, No2, Fall, pp. 37-59.

Perez L. and Dragicevic S. (2009) An agent-based approach for modeling dynamics of contagious disease spread, *International Journal of Health Geographics,* 8,50. https://doi.org/10.1186/1476-072X-8-50.

Rockett, R. J., Arnott A., Lam C. Sadsad R. Timms V. Gray K., Eden J. S., Chang S., Gall M. Draper J., Sim E., Bachmann L. N., Carter I, Basile K., Byun R., O'Sullivan, V. M., Chen, C-A. S., Maddocks S., Sorrel C. T., Dwyoer E. D., Holmes C. E., Kok J., Prokopenko M., Sintchenko V. (2020) *"Revealing COVID-19 transmission by SARS-CoV-2 Genome Sequencing and Agent Based Modeling,"* Accessed August 18. https://doi.org/10.1101/2020.04.19.048751.

Shu Teng. (2020) "Body Temperature and immunity," *Oriental Medical Care,* Mar. 26. Accessed August 18. https://orientalmedicalcare.com/2020/03/26/body-temperature-and-Immunity.

Tuomisto T. J., Yrjola J., Kolehmainen M., Bonsdorff J., Pekkanen J., Tikkanen T. (2020) *"An agent-based epidemic model REINA for COVID-19 to identify destructive policies,"* Accessed August 18. https://doi.org/10.1101/2020.04.09.20047498.

Vynnycky E. and White, R. (2010) *An Introduction to Infectious Disease Modelling,* Oxford University Press, New York.

Wilensky U. and Rand W. (2015) *An Introduction to Agent-Based Modeling,* The MIT Press, London.

Worldmeter/coronavirus_updates (2020). Accessed August 18. https://www.worldometers.info/coronavirus/country/japan/.

Biographical Sketch

Shigeaki Ogibayashi

Affiliation: Emeritus Professor, Chiba Institute of Technology

Education:

- Feb. 1992 PhD at School of Metallurgy, Tokyo University, Japan
- March 1971 Master's degree of Science, majoring in physics, School of Science, Tohoku University
- Bachelor's degree of Science, majoring in physics, Faculty of Science

Business Address: 3-5-8, Kisarazu, Chiba, Japan, 292-0802

Research and Professional Experience:

- 2017 – Present: Research on Agent-Based Modeling of Social and Economic phenomena; Emeritus Professor of Chiba Institute of Technology, Tsudanuma, Japan
- 1997-2017: Research and teaching on management science and data science, including agent-based modeling; Professor at Chiba Institute of Technology, Tsudanuma, Japan
- 1971-2017: Research and development of new technology in the field of steelmaking and solidification, especially continuous casting.

Publications from the Last 3 Years:

1. Ogibayashi S. Using agent-based modelling to understand social phenomena. *Research Outreach,* 128. doi: 10.32907/RO-128-224920 5778 (2022).
2. Ogibayashi, S. An Agent-Based Model of Infectious Diseases that Incorporates the Role of Immune Cells and Antibodies. In Yang, Z., Briesen, E. (eds.), *Proceedings of the 2020 Conference of The*

Computational Social Science Society of the Americas, pp171-201, Springer (2022).

3. Ogibayashi, S. Model structure of Agent-Based Artificial Economic System Resonsible for Reproducing Fundamental Behavior of Goods Market. In Yuji Aruka (ed.), *Digital Designs for Money, Markets, and Social Dilemmas,* pp 89-141, Springer (2022).
4. Ogibayashi, S. "Can Agent-Based Modeling Enable Scientific Policy Making Based on an Understanding of causal Mechanisms?," *Journal on Policy and Complex Systems,* Vol. 7, No1, Spring,pp. 33-39 (2021).
5. Ogibayashi, S. and Shinagawa, K. Model Structure of Agent-Based Artificial System for Reproducing the Emergence of Bullying Phenomenon, *Proceedings of the 2018 Conference of the Computational Social Science Society of the Americas,* Springer, pp229-250 (2020).
6. Ogibayashi, S. An Agent-Based Model of Infectious Diseases that Incorporates the Role of Immune Cells and Antibodies. *CSSSA 2020 Virtual Conference, Oct 8-11, 2020.* Also available at SSRN: https://ssrn.com/abstract=3665284.

Chapter 3

Endophytic Actinobacteria: A Source of Novel Bioactive Metabolites for the Treatment of Infectious Diseases

Juri Saikia[1,2], Rajkumari Mazumdar[1,3] and Debajit Thakur[1,*]

[1] Microbial Biotechnology Laboratory, Life Sciences Division,
Institute of Advanced Study in Science and Technology (IASST),
Guwahati, India
[2] Department of Biotechnology,
Gauhati University, Guwahati, India
[3] Department of Molecular Biology and Biotechnology,
Cotton University,Guwahati, India

Abstract

The emergence of infectious diseases has put on an alarming threat to human health and progress. The World Health Organization (WHO) claims that infectious diseases continue to spread and emerge and that efforts being made globally to combat newly emerging and drug resistant infections are jeopardized by a lack of new antimicrobials (2020). Covid-19, a recent pandemic that has affected the entire world and claimed the lives of 2.7 million people, has hundreds of millions of documented cases (2021).

Outbreaks of infectious disease can have detrimental social, political, and economic ramifications, and emerging and overlooking infectious diseases pose a real threat to public health. Since the historic IOM report that emphasized the significance of emerging infectious

[*] Corresponding Author's Email: debajitthakur@yahoo.co.uk.

In: Infectious Diseases
Editor: Yvette S. Brewer
ISBN: 979-8-88697-657-1

diseases, much has been taught from previous outbreaks and significant strides have been made. Yet, preparing for pandemics continues to be a significant global challenge. It has been discovered that a wide range of factors, including human behavior and activities, pathogen evolution, poverty, environmental changes, and dynamic human interactions with animals, all contributed to the emergence and spread of infectious diseases. Furthermore, the emergence of pathogens that are resistant to antibiotics has reduced the number of available treatments and caused incurable infections, necessitating the development of novel antibiotics.

There is a global need to find novel sources of antibiotics. Natural products produced by endophytic actinobacteria (EA) act as a source of potential new antibiotics. In addition, they seem to be a source of brand-new, potent compounds to fight the rising tide of pathogens with multidrug resistance. Endophytic actinobacteria reside within plant tissues and interact with the host to produce diverse bioactive metabolites. Exploration of endophytic actinobacteria from untouched ecosystems is going on in the search for new bioactive molecules. The current review highlights the isolation and discovery of potent novel bioactive metabolites produced by endophytic actinobacteria associated with diverse ecosystems.

Introduction

Infectivity describes an organism's capacity to enter, endure, and proliferate in its host, whereas infectiousness describes how easily a disease spreads to additional hosts. Physical contact, body fluids, contaminated food, objects, airborne inhalation, and vector organisms are all ways that pathogens can spread. When an infectious disease is easily transmitted by contact with an ill person or their secretions, it is referred to as contagious (e.g., influenza). Thus, an infectious disease that is particularly contagious or easily spread is referred to as a contagious disease. Other infectious/transmissible/communicable diseases with more specialized transmission modes like vector or sexual transmission, are typically not considered contagious and do not call for medical isolation (often mistakenly referred to as quarantine) of victims. Though the widespread application of the words "contagious" and "contagious disease" doesn't always respect their specific meaning (easy transmissibility) (Kumar et al., 2012).

In medicine, an infectious disease is a condition brought on by a substance, frequently a specific type of microorganism, that harms a person's health. Many times, infectious diseases can be transferred from one person to another through indirect means (like skin-to-skin contact) or direct means (e.g., via contaminated food or water). Some are transmitted by insects or other animals also. Simple infection is the invasion and replication of any number of agents in the body, including bacteria, viruses, fungi, protozoans, and worms, as well as the tissue's response to their presence or to the toxins they produce, is distinct from infectious disease (Zhang et al., 2012).

Infectious diseases are ranked as a major threat to human development and sustenance alongside war and famine. They continue to be among the prime causes of death and disability around the world. The burden of infections worldwide is significantly increased by epidemics of new and old infectious diseases that frequently appear against a background of ongoing established infections. The investigation of these novel infections reveals the characteristics of pathogenic microorganisms' evolutionary history as well as the compelling interactions between microorganisms, their hosts, and the environment (Morens et al., 2004). The causes of the rise in infectious disease incidence are not fully understood. The emergence of new infectious diseases and the resurgence of infectious diseases that were assumed to have been eradicated or controlled are thought to be influenced by changes in human demography and behavior (e.g., rising use of daycare centres, a risk factor for otitis media), technology and industry, land use and economic development (which may account for an increase in zoonotic diseases), international trade and travel, and breakdown of public health measures. For instance, since 1973, cholera, malaria, and tuberculosis have all returned or geographically spread, frequently in more severe forms. Since 1973, more than 30 new disease agents have been discovered. Since it was discovered in humans in the 1980s, *Escherichia coli* 0157 has been linked to numerous disease outbreaks and fatalities from contaminated water and food (Cassell et al., 2001).

The Uniqueness of Infectious Diseases

Infectious diseases have some distinct characteristics that set them apart from other diseases (Fauci et al., 2012):

- Potential for unforeseen and explosive global effects
- The host develops strong immunity against reinfection after recovery
- Transmissibility

- The disease is carried out by a single agent without the need for several factors
- Possible transformation into eradication
- Possibility of being preventable
- Because pathogens can reproduce and mutate, giving them a competitive evolutionary advantage over their human hosts and making them very adaptable.
- Co-evolution with or frequent derivation from other animal species
- Close reliance on the complexity and nature of human
- The potential for a treatment to have multiple beneficial effects on the microbial and animal ecosystem, as well as on preventing infection in contacts, the community, and animals.

Global Impact of Infectious Diseases

An estimated 15 million (>25%) of the 57 million annual deaths worldwide are directly related to infectious diseases. The additional millions of deaths that result from previous infections (such as streptococcal rheumatic heart disease) or complications from chronic infections, such as liver failure and hepatocellular carcinoma in people infected with hepatitis B or C viruses, are not included in this number. The recent outbreak of coronavirus disease (COVID-19) has posed a global threat to humans accounting for 6,343,783 fatalities as reported by WHO, on 7 July 2022. The World Health Organization (WHO) declared the epidemic a public health emergency of international concern on January 30, 2020 (Xiu et al., 2021). While the worldwide COVID-19 pandemic occupies everyone's attention, it's easy to overlook the other infectious diseases that can pose a threat to health, even though they still exist. In actuality, some are increasing.

Infectious diseases account for five of the top ten causes of death in the United States (pneumonia, cancer, acquired immunodeficiency syndrome (AIDS), chronic obstructive lung disease, and chronic liver disease). Between 1980 and 1992, the death rate from infectious diseases in the United States increased by 58% (the number counts only those individuals whose primary cause of death was an infectious disease). The increase was caused not only by AIDS-related deaths but also by pneumonia and septicemia in other patient populations. In addition, the prevalence of acute otitis media in children increased by 64% between 1982 and 1991, and in 1992, otitis media was the most frequently identified emergency department diagnosis (Dixon et al., 2003).

One of the top five infectious diseases worldwide is influenza (Flu), followed by sexually transmitted infections (STIs, STDs, VD), staphylococcus (Staph) infections, foodborne illnesses, and tick-borne illnesses. People living in developing countries, especially infants and children, bear the majority of the burden of morbidity (illness) and mortality brought on by infectious diseases (malaria and diarrheal illnesses alone claim the lives of about three million children each year.) In developed countries, indigenous and disadvantaged minorities are disproportionately affected by infectious disease mortality (Yuan et al., 2022).

Infectious Diseases and Antibiotic Resistance

Antibiotics are now the second most frequently prescribed class of medication. Antibiotics are now being produced at a higher rate and are becoming less expensive, leading to more applications outside the medical field. The meat industry has found that adding small amounts of antibiotics to animal feeds helps cattle, pigs, and chickens grow, which boosts sales and profits. However, this practice also has the unintended side effect of hastening the development of antibiotic resistance. Currently, non-human uses such as agriculture and aquaculture account for about 50% of all antibiotics produced globally. It is not surprising that there is a direct relationship between the amount of antibiotic use and the development of antibiotic resistance. Over the years, there has been an increase in public awareness of this issue, and many nations have mounted campaigns to inform the general public about the dangers that antibiotic-resistant bacteria pose. The Swann report, which was released in the UK in 1969, advocated for limiting the application of antibiotics in animal feedstuffs (Swann, 1969). In the Netherlands and Scandinavian nations, the use of antibiotics to upsurge animal growth has been significantly scaling down, and recent advancements are most visible. The effectiveness of these measures is evidenced by a lower rate of antibiotic resistance in farm workers and animals; however, despite these controls, resistance has not been completely eradicated and outbreaks of resistant pathogens continue to happen recurrently (Davies 2008).

Pathogenic bacteria are developing antibiotic resistance all over the world. The ability of bacteria to resist antibiotics' lethal effects is referred to as antibiotic resistance. In other words, an antibiotic that once effectively killed bacteria and treated an infection no longer does so, if at all. The infection is still active, and it could get worse. The Centers for Disease Control and Prevention (CDC) in the United States rank antibiotic resistance as one of their top public health concerns because it poses a serious threat to global health (Schinke et al., 2017). Antibiotic resistance continues to rise as a result of antibiotic overuse, and the development of new antimicrobial agents is slow. Infections with drug-resistant bacteria can result in longer and more expensive hospital stays, as well as an increased risk of death from the infection. There have been reports of dangerous resistant bacteria known as "superbugs." Over 2.8 million people get infected with antibiotic-resistant bacteria each year, with nearly 35,000 deaths. The annual cost of combating the top six multi-drug resistant bacteria in the United States exceeds $4.6 billion. Bacterial resistance is not the only type of resistance.

In 2021, cases of *Candida auris* with high resistance, which can cause severe fungal infections, were reported. Antibiotic resistance is a problem that is not just caused by humans. Resistance genes were already prevalent in the bacterial gene population much before people began using antibiotics to treat bacterial infections (Abraham & Chain, 1940). The widespread resistance to cefotaxime (CTX-M) -lactamases is an excellent illustration; it is thought that the ancestral gene was acquired from a strain of *Kluyvera* sp. and then was transferred to other bacteria (Barlow et al., 2008). Due to the indiscriminate use of specific classes of antibiotics over the past 20 years, this gene has undergone numerous mutations and gene transfers, increasing antibiotic selection, and has evolved into the family of the extended-spectrum -lactamases (ESBLs). With hundreds of different CTX-Ms being discovered in bacterial pathogens all over the world, there is currently a true pandemic. This is large-scale natural protein engineering, or what David Livermore calls "the zeitgeist of resistance" (Livermore, 2007). Despite the fact that different CTX-M genes were initially discovered in resistant bacterial strains in hospital environments, the prevalence of these genes in the general population is rising. Was this sequence of occurrences unavoidable? Was it possible to stop it? After all, ß-lactamases had been known for quite some time.

Although difficult to estimate, the costs in terms of mortality, morbidity, and economic losses are substantial. Therefore, the biggest threat today is resistant pathogens, despite the availability of a broad range of antifungal, antibacterial, and antiviral agents for most infectious diseases treatment. The development of these drug-resistant microorganisms has become a real concern (Shahbazi et al., 2018). Antibiotic-resistant bacteria now pose a serious threat to the prevention, control, and treatment of infectious diseases due to the inappropriate and arbitrary use of antibiotics as well as the baseless prescribing of antibiotics. Over 2 million Americans contract antibiotic-resistant bacteria each year in the US, which results in 35,000 fatalities. By 2050, it is predicted that more than 10 million people will die annually due to antibiotic resistance worldwide (Opoku-Temeng et al., 2019). Additionally, a growing worry is the emergence of pandrug resistance, a phenomenon in which bacteria develop resistance to all the available classes of antibiotics (Falagas et al., 2008). Therefore, new approaches, such as the discovery and development of new drugs, are needed for the prevention and control of these microorganisms.

The most promising avenue for discovering novel antibiotics, which is necessary to address the diminishing effectiveness of the currently available antibiotics, is natural product screening (Riquelme et al., 2017). For long, sources of bioactive compounds for therapeutic use have frequently included plant-associated microorganisms (Subbulakshmi et al., 2012; Abedinlou et al., 2022).

Need for a New Biocontrol Agent

New antibiotics, alternative treatments for infectious diseases, and instruments for rapid diagnosis must be found and developed in order to address the mounting issue of antibiotic resistance among pathogens. These developments will ensure the efficient and correct use of currently available antibiotics. People are losing their lives to infections that were once curable, and there is a global crisis in the treatment of infectious diseases. It is important to recognize the magnitude of this problem because, despite our best efforts, microbes continue to harm humans (Davies et al., 2008). The search for new therapeutic agents must be stepped up because microbes are both the problem and the solution to the crisis.

The future of treating infectious diseases will be determined by how the medical community, pharmaceutical industry, and academic community react in the ensuing years. The pharmaceutical industry constantly whines that the natural supply of molecules with antibiotic activity is almost depleted and that they can no longer discover useful bioactive compounds because the industry has already discovered all the readily available bioactive. It can also be explained by the inability to detect bioactive compounds when they are only present in small concentrations (Baltz, 2006). It is conceivable that developing the technology to locate overlooked compounds was not deemed necessary.

Additionally, despite having the ability to produce a huge number of bioactive small molecules, actinobacteria as a whole have been disregarded; only a small portion have been studied for therapeutic uses to date (Challis et al., 2008). Actinomycetes are a type of potential organism that is known to produce antibacterial and antifungal metabolites. Endophytic actinomycetes are being studied extensively as potential biocontrol agents around the world and are widely regarded as promising alternatives to chemical antibiotics. About two-thirds of all antibiotics that are known to exist come from actinobacteria. Almost all plants on earth contain endophytic actinobacteria, which colonize or reside within the plant tissue without harming the host plant. Endophytic actinobacteria invade the host plant through the roots and spread to other areas (Almaary et al., 2021).

Living organisms produce a large number (over one million) of diverse metabolites. Most of these metabolites have been discovered in plants, however, microorganisms are particularly abundant sources of more than 20,000 biologically active substances that affect the functionality and survival of other organisms. Secondary metabolites have no known specific function in the primary metabolism of organisms, but their huge diversity represents the biological role of organisms in their environment, particularly in interactions between organisms, and demonstrates their relevance as toxins and signals. The genomic revolution has made it abundantly clear that our understanding of the structures and occurrence of bacterial metabolites is far from saturated, despite the recent decline in the rate of discovery of active metabolites (such as antibiotics) (Baltz et al., 2008). Even the genomes of well-known bacteria have uncovered genes that may be responsible for the synthesis of previously undiscovered metabolites, and it is thought that the metabolites discovered so far only make up a small portion of the entire metabolic repertoire (Walsh et al., 2010; Traxler et al., 2012). The fact that only a small portion of bacteria have been successfully cultivated to date makes it seem unlikely that the metabolic potential of bacteria will ever be fully understood (Brader et al., 2014).

Microbes that lived inside living plant tissues without causing any disease or significant morphological changes are known as endophytes. Endophytes are known as a reservoir of bioactive metabolites and plants hosts diverse group of endophytes. Out of these actinobacteria has been proven to be a major phylum and the majority of these bioactive compounds are extracted from actinobacteria, primarily from the well-studied genus *Streptomyces*. *Streptomyces* is the most thoroughly studied microbial genus for secondary metabolite production (Demain et al., 2009; Miao et al., 2010). They have untapped potential for the development of bioactive agents for therapeutic use. Human health and well-being are seriously threatened by harsh agrochemicals and drug-resistant pathogens.

The most promising approach to addressing these two issues is to use beneficial microorganisms and their metabolic inventions. Large biologically active metabolites from numerous microorganisms, particularly actinomycetes, have been found since the 1940s when penicillin and streptomycin were first discovered. A lot of attention has been paid to actinomycetes recently because of their diverse metabolic potential with applications in agriculture, medicine, and industry. These organisms were also searched from unexplored, undeveloped ecosystems. Endophytic actinomycetes that reside in living plant tissues are recognized as a potential hub for novel bioactive substances for drug-lead discovery. There is a chance that more study of the endophytic actinomycetes that live on plants will lead to the discovery of new taxa and their metabolites, which could have biotechnological significance (Masand et al., 2015).

Endophytic Actinobacteria as A Source of Bioactive Metabolites

Actinobacteria are gram-positive microbes with bacterial and fungal cell morphologies (aerial and substrate mycelium). According to Petrini in 1991, the Greek words "atakis" (array) and "mykes" (fungus) were used to create the term "actinomycetes." 45% of the antibiotics produced by actinobacteria came from various *Streptomyces* sp. The presence of high G C in their genome is thought to be a major attribute for the ability to produce diverse active metabolites. Soil, water, sediments, and plants, are commonly reported substrates for actinobacteria isolation. De Bary 1886 first introduced the term endophyte for microorganisms (bacteria, fungi, and yeast) colonizing internal plant tissues. Endophytes were defined by Petrini in 1991 as any organism that colonizes internal plant tissue at some point in its life cycle without any apparent damage to the host plant. There is evidence that endophytes support plant growth, shield against pathogens, and maintain a co-evolutionary mechanism with other species.

The use of antibiotics without an understanding of dosage during medical procedures, as well as their release into the environment as a result of anthropogenic activities, causes pathogens to adapt and become resistant, resulting in lethal infections against human health (Sungthong and Nakaew, 2014). Alternatively, excessive use of chemical fungicides in agricultural practices has a negative impact on the environment and human health (Muri et al., 2009; Bozdogan, 2014). Due to these obstacles, a focused search for new microorganisms with bioactive metabolites for potential interdisciplinary applications to safeguard the environment and human health is ongoing. While a sizable pool of useful dynamic microorganisms has already been explored and isolated from a variety of natural habitats around the world, endophytes, which colonize the interior tissues of host plants, have received limited attention and are being investigated as a potential source of antibiotics. Endophytic bioactive substances aid the host plant to grow systemic resistance against harmful pathogens. These substances are also extensively used as antibiotic, anti-viral, and anti-cancer agents in pharmaceutical industries (Guo et al., 2008).

Endophytes (actinomycetes, fungi, and bacteria) play important roles in the synthesis of bioactive compounds. Bioactive peptides, alkaloids, steroids, terpenoids, flavonoids, polyketones, phenols, and quinols are examples of bioactive compounds. The natural insecticide azadirachtin, which is produced by endophytes has been discovered applications in agriculture, industry, and medicine (Molina et al., 2012). Endophytic actinomycetes are one of the promising sources of bioactive agents that can be used to protect crops and develop therapeutic agents (Prashith Kekuda, 2016). There are currently over 140 genera of actinomycetes that have been identified, but only a handful of these genera are known to have produced the mass of the known essential antibiotics (Pimentel-Elardo et al., 2010). A variety of secondary metabolites that are produced by actinomycetes have the potential to become therapeutic agents because they exhibit biological activity. Untapped sources of novel secondary metabolites can be found in marine actinomycetes (Lam, 2006). Significant antibacterial activity was demonstrated by *Streptomyces rochei* CH1, an endophytic actinomycete of *Cinnamomum* sp., against a variety of test pathogens, including *Vibrio parahemolyticus, Aeromonas caviae* and *Pseudomonas aeruginosa* (Roy and Banerjee, 2015). Broad spectrum antimicrobial activities against *Escherichia coli* MTCC 739, *Candida albicans* MTCC 3017, *Micrococcus luteus* NCIM 2170, *P. aeruginosa* MTCC 2453, and *P. aeruginosa* was exhibited by *Streptomyces cyaneofuscatus* (KY-287599)

From endophytic *S. fradiae*, various antimicrobial, anti-inflammatory, and anticancer compounds have been reported. From the roots of *Zingiber officinale* and *Alpinia galanga*, Taechowisan and Lumyong (2003) isolated 59 endophytic *Streptomyces* species with strong bioactivities against pathogens *Colletotrichum musae* and *Candida albicans*. Similar to this, *Streptomyces* sp. from maize was found to have antimicrobial properties against a variety of bacterial and fungal pathogens by Araujo et al., in 2000. The antimicrobial effects of endophytic *Streptomyces* sp. against *P. fluorescence* from *Azadirachta indica* were investigated by Verma et al., (2009). The peptide antibiotic coronamycin, which has activity against *Cryptococcus neoformans* and *Plasmodium falciparum*, is produced by an endophytic *Streptomyces* species from monster species plants (Ezra et al., 2004).

Bafilomycin family member 24-demethylbafilomycin C1 was produced by endophytic *Streptomyces* sp. CS and is used to treat pediatric B cell acute lymphoblastic leukaemia by targeting the autophagy and apoptosis pathways (Li et al., 2010; Qin et al., 2011; Yuan et al., 2015). Two new novobiocin analogs and two new cedarmycins were produced by endophytic *Streptomyces* sp. obtained from *Aucuba japonica* and *Cryptomeria japonica*, respectively. Alnumycin, a brand-new naphthoquinone antibiotic, was also discovered in *Streptomyces* sp., an endophytic strain from *Alnus glutinosa*. An endophyte of the snake vine plant called *Streptomyces* sp. NRRL30562 produced the novel peptide antibiotic munumbicins A-D40, which exhibits broad-spectrum antimicrobial activity against a number of human diseases as well as phytopathogenic fungi and bacteria. Kakadumycin, which is chemically related to echinomycin, was produced by endophytic *Streptomyces* sp. NRRL30566 was extracted from a fern-leaved grevillea (*Grevillea pteridifolia*) tree (Castillo et al., 2003).

Many novel antibiotics developed in recent years, from medicinal plant-derived endophytic actinobacteria displayed activity at much lower concentrations. This proves that the antibiotics made from endophytic actinobacteria, primarily those of the genus *Streptomyces*, have potent and versatile microbiocidal properties. Out of 65 strains, 12 strains of endophytic actinobacteria, primarily *Streptomyces* from *Paeonia lactiflora*, *Achyranthes bidentata*, *Artemisia argyi* and *Radix platycodi* were able to inhibit penicillin-resistant *Staphylococcus aureus*, belonging to the genus *Glycomyces* (Zhang et al., 2012). According to a study by Wang et al. (2014), perlolyrine, 1-hydroxy-b-carboline, lumichrome, and 1H-indole-3-carboxaldehyde from *Jishengella endophytica* had modest antiviral activity against influenza virus type A subtype H1N1 with IC50 values of 38.3, 25.0, 39.7, and 45.9 lg ml-1, respectively. Furthermore, they hypothesized that 1-hydroxy-b-carboline might be a promising new anti-H1N1 drug breakthrough.

According to Tanvir et al., (2014), endophytic *Streptomyces* sp. with larvicidal activity include strains obtained from *Echinops spinosus, Artemisia herbaalba, Mentha longifolia and Balotla andulate* (2008). *Streptomyces* sp. an endophyte, was found in *Citrus aurantifolia* plants from various indian growing regions. Low concentrations of lerdarmycins A and B isolated from *Streptomyces* sp. TP A0456 were effective against fungi. Sedamycin, derived from *Streptomyces* sp. heduya-48 is one of the new compounds that had activities against clinical dermatophytes (El-Gendy and EL-Bondkly 2010). Actinomycin D with antifungal activity was extracted by Taechowisan and Lumyong in 2008 from *Streptomyces* sp. TCO22.

Castillo et al., (2002) reported the broad-spectrum activity of purified munambicins E4, E5, and A-D from endophytic *Streptomyces* against both gram-positive and negative bacterial pathogens. According to Mustafa et al., (2016), the isolate *S. cyaneofuscutus* KY287599 demonstrated broad-spectrum activity against *C. albicans* MTCC3017, S. aureus MTCC 3160, *Escherichia coli* MTCC739, and *Micrococcus luleus* NCIM 2170. *Geotrichum candidum* was resistant to the antimicrobial effects of *Streptomyces* sp. TQR12-4 (Hong-Thao et al., 2016). *Streptomyces* sp. derived from *Kennedia nigriscans* stem was reported to have munumbicins A, B, C, and D possessing antimalarial activity (Castillo et al., 2002). D was the most potent of the four types against *P. falciparum. S. albidoflavus* antimycin A 18, which was obtained from mangrove plants, exhibited potent action against human pathogens (Yan et al., 2010).

According to Shiomi et al., (2005), *Streptomyces* sp. K01-0031 produced antimycin 1-7, which belongs to the family of bicyclic chromopeptide lactones and inhibits transcription. The novel peptide antibiotic coronomycin from *Streptomyces* sp. MSU2110 isolated from *Monstera* sp. was described as having activity against *P. falciparum* and *C. neoformans* (Joseph et al., 2012). Cyclopentenone extracted from *Streptomyces* sp. associated with *Aegiceras corniculatum* has valuable applications in the pharmaceutical industry (Lin et al., 2008).

In the broth culture of *Streptomyces* sp. TC052 from *Alpinia galanga*, two antimicrobial compounds, isocutellarin and cichoriin, were discovered, which were found to be effective against both gram-positive and gram-negative bacteria as well as yeast cells (Taechowisan et al., 2007, 2008). 17 actinobacteria strains isolated from Antarctica were found to have secondary metabolites with potential antitumor effects. Brown algae-derived *Streptomyces sundarbansensis* WR1L1S8 yields a novel anti-MRSA compound, [2-hydroxy-5-((6-hydroxy-4-oxo-4H-pyran-2-yl) methyl)-2-propylchroman-4-one], which is selectively active against the gram-positive pathogenic MRSA with a MIC of 6 lL, along with three other known polyketides, phaphaeochromycin B, phaeochromycin C and phaeochromycin E (Djinni et al., 2013, 2014). Two new bafilomycins belonging to macrolide group antibiotics namely 29-hydroxybafilomycin D and 9-hydroxy-bafilomycin D were extracted from *Streptomyces* sp. YIM56209 was obtained from the stems of *Drymaria cordata* (Li et al., 2015). The first naturally occurring antimycin, known as Antimycin A18, was discovered in endophytic *Streptomyces* albidoflavus I07A-01824, associated with the leaves of the mangrove plant *Bruguiera gymnorrhiza* (Yan et al., 2010). A B-carboline, 1-vinyl-b-carboline-3-carboxylic acid active against both bacteria and fungi was isolated from endophytic actinomycete *Microbispora* sp. LGMB259 (Savi et al., 2015).

In addition to isolating 320 endophytic actinobacterial strains from Taklamakan Desert psammophytes, Wang et al., 2021 also recognised 3 strains as new species and 16 strains as potential new taxa. Two new streptogramin-type antibiotics, acetyl-griseoviridin and desulphurizing griseoviridin, as well as the more well-known griseoviridin, were discovered to be produced by one strain, 8P21H-1, with subtantial antibacterial activity. The major bottleneck of the rediscovery of well-known antibiotics was addressed in this study, which established a valuable integrated strategy for tracing new and/or bioactive compounds. It also helped in the discovery of novel secondary metabolites.

Mahdi et al., 2022 first reported endophytic actinobacteria from *Luffa cylindrica* and showed strong antagonistic activity against *S. aureus*, *P. aeruginosa*, and *E. coli*. Three strains, KUMS-B3, KUMS-B4, and KUMS-B6, were identified as endophytes for the first time. According to the study, the isolated strains from Luffa produce a wide range of bioactive compounds that could be used as new sources for drug candidates to treat infections. Six endophytic actinobacteria from *Citrullus colocynthis* were examined, identified, and their antimicrobial activity was evaluated for the first time (Ali et al., 2022). For the first time, three of them were described as endophytes. The stain KUMS-C6 displayed the broadest spectrum of antibacterial activity against all test bacteria, while five strains demonstrated antagonist activity against *S. aureus*, *P. aeruginosa*, and *E. coli*.

Beilunmycin, a new virginiamycins antibiotic (1), and three known virginiamycin antibiotics, 16-hydroxy-virginiamycin M1 (2), virginiamycin M2 (3), and virginiamycin M1 (4), were reported from the culture of a mangrove-derived endophytic *Streptomyces* sp. 2BBP-J2 by Jiang et al., 2020.

Ahmed et al., 2022 found significant antimicrobial activity of actinomycetes extracts against multidrug-resistant *Staphylococcus aureus* and *Salmonella* spp. isolated from meat.

Peptides called complestatins were produced by *Streptomyces lavendulae*. These peptides act by interacting with the target cells' surface molecules and inhibit the adsorption of HIV-1 (human immunodeficiency virus type 1) to the cells, but they did not exhibit inhibitory activity against HIV enzymes (Salim et al., 2021). From the culture supernatants of *Streptomyces chromofuscus* protease inhibitor (PISC-2002) was reported. In the fight against the influenza virus A/Rostock/34, PISC-2002 is crucial (Angelova et al., 2006). The discovery and production of antiviral metabolites by endophytes have become a hot topic in the development of viral therapeutics and antiviral drugs. The production of CoV vaccines is ongoing in an effort to lower the incidence of virally transmitted diseases. Endophytic microbes are rich in natural bioactive substances that have the potential to act as immunomodulators and protease inhibitors (Okoye et al., 2015). They have demonstrated great promise as potential recipients of complementary and alternative medicine or antiviral medications for the prevention and treatment of CoVs (Naik 2019; Suwannarach et al., 2020;).

Numerous endophytic bioactive substances have had their anti-coronavirus properties studied (2021). Anti-CoVs substances like dimethyl asterriquinone D, ganolucidic acid A, ganoderic acid A, ganoderiol acid B, and colossolactone A, E, G, and V were isolated using endophytes. Additionally, the anti-HIV and anti-cancer effects of these substances were thoroughly studied. *Streptomyces misionensis* MI22 obtained from *Madhuca insignis Radlk.*, from Western Ghats of India demonstarted a broad spectrum anti-microbial activity against MRSA (methicillin-resistant *Staphylococcus aureus* (25.00 ± 1.00 mm) followed by *Bacillus subtilis* (23.66 ± 0.57 mm), *Escherichia coli* (22.00 ± 0.00 mm), and *Candida albicans* (18.00 ± 0.00 mm) (Mondal et al., 2021) and suggested that this strain could be a lead for novel bioactive metabolites against multidrug-resistant pathogens. The trehangelins, which are composed of two trehalose molecules and an angelic acid, were obtained from *Polymorphospora rubra* K07-0510, the actinoallolides, 12-membered macrolides, from *Actinoallomurus fulvus* MK10-036, and the spoxazomicins, pyochelin family antibiotics, from *Streptosporangium oxazolinicum* K07-0460T (Matsumoto et al., 2017). Dodecanoic acid, dl-alanyl-l-leucine, and phenyl propanedioic acid are three potential inhibitors of New Delhi metallo-lactamase-1 that were discovered by Cheepurupalli et al. in 2021 in endophytic *Streptomyces* sp.

Conclusion and Future Prospects

> The world has forgotten how important it is to fight disease and improve health in order to reduce poverty. Infectious diseases are a serious social problem that now affects both the health of the individual and the health of the environment in which we live. We must acknowledge them as a shared threat that has been long ignored at great cost and come together as a world to fight them.

The emergence of bacteria that are resistant to antibiotics has reduced available therapies and resulted in infections that are incurable, necessitating the development of novel antibiotics to battle against bacteria. Antimicrobial resistance is a persistent problem that has been addressed in a number of ways. The therapeutic arsenal is being strengthened and expanded by the creation of novel classes of antibiotic, antiparasitic and antiviral agents directed at different microbial targets, frequently with the help of high-throughput compound screening. Endophytic actinobacteria (EA) natural products act as a source of potential new antibiotics.

As our understanding of these organisms advances, the potential to utilize endophytic bacteria's unique capacities to synthesize bioactive compounds, either independently or in cooperation with plants, is increasing every day. It is still largely unknown how endophytes affect plant physiology and metabolism and how they utilize the intermediate products of primary and secondary metabolism as food and precursors to either generate new compounds or improve the already-existing significant secondary metabolites. The development of pharmaceutical products have a long history of using natural products in a safe and effective manner. Mining under or unexplored habitats, the future of new antibiotic developments against diseases with multi-drug resistance pathogens looks bright.

References

Abedinlou, H., Bahrami, Y., Mohammadi, S., & Kakaei, E. (2022). Rare actinobacteria and their potential biotechnological applications. Sci. J. Kurdistan Univ. *Med. Sci*, 26(7), 108-131.

Abraham, E. P., & Chain, E. (1940). An enzyme from bacteria able to destroy penicillin. *Nature*, 146(3713), 837-837.

Ahmed, W., Helal, I., Zaky, M., & Abdulla, H. M. (2022). Antimicrobial Activity of Actinomycetes Extracts against Multidrug-Resistant Staphylococcus aureus and

Salmonella spp. isolated from meat. *Alfarama Journal of Basic & Applied Sciences*, 3(2), 283-299.

Ali, A. R., Bahrami, Y., Kakaei, E., Mohammadzadeh, S., Bouk, S., & Jalilian, N. (2022). Isolation and identification of endophytic actinobacteria from Citrullus colocynthis (L.) Schrad and their antibacterial properties. *Microbial Cell Factories*, 21(1), 1-17.

Almaary, K. S., Alharbi, N. S., Kadaikunnan, S., Khaled, J. M., Rajivgandhi, G., Ramachandran, G., & Manoharan, N. (2021). Anti-bacterial effect of marine sea grasses mediated endophytic actinomycetes against K. pneumoniae. *Journal of King Saud University-Science*, 33(6), 101528.

Angelova, L., Dalgalarrondo, M., Minkov, I., Danova, S., Kirilov, N., Serkedjieva, J., & Ivanova, I. (2006). Purification and characterisation of a protease inhibitor from Streptomyces chromofuscus 34-1 with an antiviral activity. *Biochimica et Biophysica Acta (BBA)-General Subjects,* 1760(8), 1210-1216.

Araújo, M. B., & Williams, P. H. (2000). Selecting areas for species persistence using occurrence data. *Biological Conservation*, 96(3), 331-345.

Baltz, R. H. (2006). Marcel Faber Roundtable: is our antibiotic pipeline unproductive because of starvation, constipation or lack of inspiration? *Journal of Industrial Microbiology and Biotechnology*, 33(7), 507-513.

Baltz, R. H. (2008). Renaissance in antibacterial discovery from actinomycetes. *Current Opinion in Pharmacology*, *8*(5), 557-563.

Barlow, G., Nathwani, D., Myers, E., Sullivan, F., Stevens, N., Duffy, R., & Davey, P. (2008). Identifying barriers to the rapid administration of appropriate antibiotics in community-acquired pneumonia. *Journal of Antimicrobial Chemotherapy*, *61*(2), 442-451.

Bozdogan, A. M. (2014). Assessment of total risk on non-target organisms in fungicide application for agricultural sustainability. *Sustainability*, 6(2), 1046-1058.

Brader, G., Compant, S., Mitter, B., Trognitz, F., & Sessitsch, A. (2014). Metabolic potential of endophytic bacteria. *Current Opinion in Biotechnology*, *27*, 30-37.

Cassell, G. H., & Mekalanos, J. (2001). Development of antimicrobial agents in the era of new and reemerging infectious diseases and increasing antibiotic resistance. *JAMA*, 285(5), 601-605.

Castillo, U. F., Strobel, G. A., Ford, E. J., Hess, W. M., Porter, H., Jensen, J. B., & Yaver, D. (2002). Munumbicins, wide-spectrum antibiotics produced by Streptomyces NRRL 30562, endophytic on Kennedia nigriscansaaThe GenBank accession number for the sequence determined in this work is AY127079. *Microbiology,* 148(9), 2675-2685.

Castillo, U., Harper, J. K., Strobel, G. A., Sears, J., Alesi, K., Ford, E., & Teplow, D. (2003). Kakadumycins, novel antibiotics from Streptomyces sp. NRRL 30566, an endophyte of Grevillea pteridifolia. *FEMS Microbiology Letters*, 224(2), 183-190.

Challis, G. L. (2008). Mining microbial genomes for new natural products and biosynthetic pathways. *Microbiology*, 154(6), 1555-1569.

Cheepurupalli, L., Diaz, A., Gopal, A. C., Rathore, S. S., Ramakrishnan, V., & Ramakrishnan, J. (2021). In vitro and in silico screening of Klebsiella pneumoniae new Delhi metallo-β-lactamase-1 inhibitors from endophytic *Streptomyces spp. Journal of Biomolecular Structure and Dynamics*, 1-13.

Davies, J. (2008). Resistance redux: infectious diseases, antibiotic resistance and the future of mankind. *EMBO reports*, 9(S1), S18-S21.

Demain, A. L., & Sanchez, S. (2009). Microbial drug discovery: 80 years of progress. *The Journal of Antibiotics*, 62(1), 5-16.

Dixon, A. R. (2003). *Health and wealth: Dietary supplements, network marketing and the commodification of health*. University of Hawai'i at Manoa.

Djinni, I., Defant, A., Kecha, M., & Mancini, I. (2013). Antibacterial polyketides from the marine alga-derived endophitic Streptomyces sundarbansensis: a study on hydroxypyrone tautomerism. *Marine Drugs*, 11(1), 124-135.

Djinni, I., Defant, A., Kecha, M., & Mancini, I. (2014). Metabolite profile of marine-derived endophytic S treptomyces sundarbansensis WR 1 L 1 S 8 by liquid chromatography–mass spectrometry and evaluation of culture conditions on antibacterial activity and mycelial growth. *Journal of Applied Microbiology*, *116*(1), 39-50.

El-Gendy, M. M., & El-Bondkly, A. M. (2010). Production and genetic improvement of a novel antimycotic agent, saadamycin, against dermatophytes and other clinical fungi from endophytic Streptomyces sp. Hedaya48. *Journal of Industrial Microbiology and Biotechnology*, 37(8), 831-841.

Ezra, D., Castillo, U. F., Strobel, G. A., Hess, W. M., Porter, H., Jensen, J. B., & Yaver, D. (2004). Coronamycins, peptide antibiotics produced by a verticillate Streptomyces sp.(MSU-2110) endophytic on Monstera sp. *Microbiology,* 150(4), 785-793.

Falagas, M. E., & Karageorgopoulos, D. E. (2008). Pandrug resistance (PDR), extensive drug resistance (XDR), and multidrug resistance (MDR) among Gram-negative bacilli: need for international harmonization in terminology. *Clinical Infectious Diseases*, 46(7), 1121-1122.

Guo, B., Wang, Y., Sun, X., & Tang, K. (2008). Bioactive natural products from endophytes: a review. *Applied Biochemistry and Microbiology*, 44(2), 136-142.

Hong-Thao, P. T., Mai-Linh, N. V., Hong-Lien, N. T., & Van Hieu, N. (2016). Biological characteristics and antimicrobial activity of endophytic Streptomyces sp. TQR12-4 isolated from elite Citrus nobilis cultivar Ham Yen of Vietnam. *International Journal of Microbiology,* 2016.

Jiang, Z. K., Hu, X. X., Xiao, L. L., Ren, Y. R., Shakhtina, A. N., Lukianov, D. A., & Sun, C. H. (2021). Beilunmycin, a new virginiamycins antibiotic from mangrove-derived Streptomyces sp. 2BBP-J2 and the antibacterial activity by inhibiting protein translation. *Journal of Asian Natural Products Research*, 23(10), 992-1000.

Joseph, B., Sankarganesh, P., Edwin, B. T., & Raj, S. J. (2012). Endophytic streptomycetes from plants with novel green chemistry: review. *Int. J. Biol. Chem*, *6*, 42-52.

Kumar, S. V., Damodar, G., Ravikanth, S., & Vijayakumar, G. (2012). *An Overview on Infectious Disease*.

Lam, K. S. (2006). Discovery of novel metabolites from marine actinomycetes. *Current Opinion in Microbiology*, 9(3), 245-251.

Li, J., Lu, C., & Shen, Y. (2010). Macrolides of the bafilomycin family produced by Streptomyces sp. CS. *The Journal of Antibiotics,* 63(10), 595-599.

Lin, Z. J., Lu, X. M., Zhu, T. J., Fang, Y. C., Gu, Q. Q., & Zhu, W. (2008). GPR12 Selections of the metabolites from an endophytic Streptomyces sp. asociated with Cistanches deserticola. *Archives of Pharmacal Research*, 31(9), 1108-1114.

Livermore, D. M., Canton, R., Gniadkowski, M., Nordmann, P., Rossolini, G. M., Arlet, G., & Woodford, N. (2007). CTX-M: changing the face of ESBLs in Europe. *Journal of Antimicrobial Chemotherapy*, 59(2), 165-174.

Mahdi, R. A., Bahrami, Y., & Kakaei, E. (2022). Identification and antibacterial evaluation of endophytic actinobacteria from Luffa cylindrica. *Scientific Reports*, 12(1), 1-13.

Masand, M., Jose, P. A., Menghani, E., & Jebakumar, S. R. D. (2015). Continuing hunt for endophytic actinomycetes as a source of novel biologically active metabolites. *World Journal of Microbiology and Biotechnology*, 31(12), 1863-1875.

Matsumoto, A., & Takahashi, Y. (2017). Endophytic actinomycetes: promising source of novel bioactive compounds. *The Journal of Antibiotics*, 70(5), 514-519.

Miao, V., & Davies, J. (2010). Actinobacteria: the good, the bad, and the ugly. *Antonie Van Leeuwenhoek*, 98(2), 143-150.

Molina, G., Pimentel, M. R., Bertucci, T. C., & Pastore, G. M. (2012). Application of fungal endophytes in biotechnological processes. *Chem. Eng. Trans*, 27.

Mondal, S., & Ravishankar Rai, V. (2021). Molecular profiling and anti-infective potency of endophytic actinomycetes inhabiting Madhuca insignis Radlk., from Western Ghats of India. *Journal of Genetic Engineering and Biotechnology*, *19*(1), 1-10.

Morens, D. M., Folkers, G. K., & Fauci, A. S. (2004). The challenge of emerging and re-emerging infectious diseases. *Nature*, *430*(6996), 242-249.

Muri, S. D., van der Voet, H., Boon, P. E., van Klaveren, J. D., & Brüschweiler, B. J. (2009). Comparison of human health risks resulting from exposure to fungicides and mycotoxins via food. *Food and Chemical Toxicology*, 47(12), 2963-2974.

Mustafa, S., Lakshmi, D. V., Syed, R., Sekhar, C. C., Sahoo, B. K., Surendrababu, M. S., & Kumar, C. G. (2016). Synthesis, antimicrobial, bactericidal and anti-biofilm activities of novel pyridyl tetrazole analogs. *J Chem Pharm Res*, 8(11), 1-6.

Okoye, F. B., Nworu, C. S., Debbab, A., Esimone, C. O., & Proksch, P. (2015). Two new cytochalasins from an endophytic fungus, KL-1.1 isolated from Psidium guajava leaves. *Phytochemistry Letters*, 14, 51-55.

Opoku-Temeng, C., Kobayashi, S. D., & DeLeo, F. R. (2019). Klebsiella pneumoniae capsule polysaccharide as a target for therapeutics and vaccines. *Computational and Structural Biotechnology Journal*, 17, 1360-1366.

Petrini, O. (1991). Fungal endophytes of tree leaves. In *Microbial Ecology of Leaves* (pp. 179-197). Springer, New York, NY.

Pimentel-Elardo, S. M., Kozytska, S., Bugni, T. S., Ireland, C. M., Moll, H., & Hentschel, U. (2010). Anti-parasitic compounds from Streptomyces sp. strains isolated from Mediterranean sponges. *Marine Drugs,* 8(2), 373-380.

Prashith-Kekuda, T. R. (2016). Isolation, characterization and antimicrobial potential of endophytic actinomycetes. *Int J Curr Microbiol Appl Sci*, 5(57), 100-116.

Qin, S., Xing, K., Jiang, J. H., Xu, L. H., & Li, W. J. (2011). Biodiversity, bioactive natural products and biotechnological potential of plant-associated endophytic actinobacteria. *Applied Microbiology and Biotechnology*, 89(3), 457-473.

Riquelme, C., Enes Dapkevicius, M. D. L., Miller, A. Z., Charlop-Powers, Z., Brady, S., Mason, C., & Cheeptham, N. (2017). Biotechnological potential of Actinobacteria from Canadian and Azorean volcanic caves. *Applied Microbiology and Biotechnology*, 101(2), 843-857.

Roy, S., & Banerjee, D. (2015). Bioactive endophytic actinomycetes of Cinnamomum sp.; isolation, identification, activity guided purification and process optimization of active metabolite. *American Journal of Microbiology*, 6(1), 4.

Savi, D. C., Shaaban, K. A., Vargas, N., Ponomareva, L. V., Possiede, Y. M., Thorson, J. S., & Rohr, J. (2015). Microbispora sp. LGMB259 endophytic actinomycete isolated from Vochysia divergens (Pantanal, Brazil) producing β-carbolines and indoles with biological activity. *Current Microbiology*, *70*(3), 345-354.

Schinke, C., Martins, T., Queiroz, S. C., Melo, I. S., & Reyes, F. G. (2017). Antibacterial compounds from marine bacteria, 2010–2015. *Journal of Natural Products*, 80(4), 1215-1228.

Shahbazi, S., Karam, M. R. A., Habibi, M., Talebi, A., & Bouzari, S. (2018). Distribution of extended-spectrum β-lactam, quinolone, and carbapenem resistance genes, and genetic diversity among uropathogenic Escherichia coli isolates in Tehran, Iran. *Journal of Global Antimicrobial Resistance*, 14, 118-125.

Shankar Naik, B. (2019). Developments in taxol production through endophytic fungal biotechnology: a review. *Oriental Pharmacy and Experimental Medicine*, 19(1), 1-13.

Shiomi, K., Hatae, K., Hatano, H., Matsumoto, A., Takahashi, Y., Jiang, C. L., & Ōmura, S. (2005). A new antibiotic, antimycin A9, produced by Streptomyces sp. K01-0031. *The Journal of Antibiotics*, 58(1), 74-78.

Subbulakshmi, G. K., Thalavaipandian, A., Ramesh, V., & Rajendran, A. (2012). Bioactive endophytic fungal isolates of Biota orientalis (L) Endl., Pinus excelsa Wall and Thuja occidentalis L. *International Journal of Advanced Life Sciences* (IJALS), 4, 9-15.

Sungthong, R., & Nakaew, N. (2015). The genus Nonomuraea: a review of a rare actinomycete taxon for novel metabolites. *Journal of Basic Microbiology*, 55(5), 554-565.

Suwannarach, N., Kumla, J., Sujarit, K., Pattananandecha, T., Saenjum, C., & Lumyong, S. (2020). Natural bioactive compounds from fungi as potential candidates for protease inhibitors and immunomodulators to apply for coronaviruses. *Molecules,* 25(8), 1800.

Taechowisan, T., Chuaychot, N., Chanaphat, S., Wanbanjob, A., & Shen, Y. (2008). Biological activity of chemical constituents isolated from Streptomyces sp. Tc052, an endophyte in Alpinia galanga. *Int J Pharmacol*, 4(2), 95-101.

Taechowisan, T., Lu, C., Shen, Y., & Lumyong, S. (2007). Antitumor activity of 4-arylcoumarins from endophytic Streptomyces aureofaciens CMUAc130. *Journal of Cancer Research and Therapeutics*, 3(2), 86.

Taechowisan, T., & Lumyong, S. (2003). Activity of endophytic actimomycetes from roots of Zingiber officinale and Alpinia galanga against phytopathogenic fungi. *Annals of Microbiology,* 53(3), 291-298.

Tanvir, R., Sajid, I., & Hasnain, S. (2014). Larvicidal potential of Asteraceae family endophytic actinomycetes against Culex quinquefasciatus mosquito larvae. *Natural Product Research*, 28(22), 2048-2052.

Traxler, M. F., & Kolter, R. (2012). A massively spectacular view of the chemical lives of microbes. *Proceedings of the National Academy of Sciences*, 109(26), 10128-10129.

Verma, V. C., Gond, S. K., Kumar, A., Mishra, A., Kharwar, R. N., & Gange, A. C. (2009). Endophytic actinomycetes from Azadirachta indica A. Juss.: isolation, diversity, and anti-microbial activity. *Microbial Ecology*, 57(4), 749-756.

Walsh, C. T., & Fischbach, M. A. (2010). Natural products version 2.0: connecting genes to molecules. *Journal of the American Chemical Society*, 132(8), 2469-2493.

Wang, P., Kong, F., Wei, J., Wang, Y., Wang, W., Hong, K., & Zhu, W. (2014). Alkaloids from the mangrove-derived actinomycete Jishengella endophytica 161111. *Marine Drugs*, 12(1), 477-490.

Wang, T., Li, F., Lu, Q., Wu, G., Jiang, Z., Liu, S., & Sun, C. (2021). Diversity, novelty, antimicrobial activity, and new antibiotics of cultivable endophytic actinobacteria isolated from psammophytes collected from Taklamakan Desert. *Journal of Pharmaceutical Analysis,* 11(2), 241-250.

Xiu, X., Wang, A., Qian, Q., & Wu, S. (2021). The US Public's Perception of the Threat of COVID-19 During the Rapid Spread of the COVID-19 Outbreak: Cross-Sectional Survey Study. *Journal of Medical Internet Research, 23*(2), e23400.

Yan, L. L., Han, N. N., Zhang, Y. Q., Yu, L. Y., Chen, J., Wei, Y. Z., & Sun, C. H. (2010). Antimycin A18 produced by an endophytic Streptomyces albidoflavus isolated from a mangrove plant. *The Journal of Antibiotics*, 63(5), 259-261.

Yuan, K., Huang, X. L., Yan, W., Zhang, Y. X., Gong, Y. M., Su, S. Z., & Lu, L. (2022). A systematic review and meta-analysis on the prevalence of stigma in infectious diseases, including COVID-19: a call to action. *Molecular Psychiatry*, 27(1), 19-33.

Yuan, N., Song, L., Zhang, S., Lin, W., Cao, Y., Xu, F., & Wang, J. (2015). Bafilomycin A1 targets both autophagy and apoptosis pathways in pediatric B-cell acute lymphoblastic leukemia. *Haematologica*, 100(3), 345.

Zhang, X., Ren, K., & Zhang, L. (2012). Screening and preliminary identification of medicinal plants endophytic actinomycetes used for inhibiting penicillin-resistant Staphylococcus aureus. *International Journal of Biology*.

Biographical Sketches

Debajit Thakur

Affiliation: Institute of Advanced Study in Science and Technology (IASST)

Education: Academic qualification from Bachelor's degree onwards.

- 2004: PhD in Life Sciences (Applied Microbiology)from Dibrugarh University, Assam*

- 1998: M.Sc. in Botany (Specialization in Microbiology) from Cotton College, Guwahati, Gauhati University, Guwahati, Assam
- 1995: B.Sc. in Botany (Major), Chemistry, Zoology from Sibsagar College, Sibsagar Dibrugarh University, Assam

*Ph.D. research work supervised by Dr. M. K. Roy (Retd. Head & Sc. F) Biotechnology Division, North East Institute of Science & Technology (CSIR), Jorhat, Assam. Thesis title: "Heterokaryosis of *Streptomyces* sp. for improved biotransformation of penicillin to cephalexin with simultaneous production of an antibiotic."

Business Address: Institute of Advanced Study in Science and Technology, Garchuk, Paschim Boragaon, Vigyan Path, Guwahati- 781035, Assam, India

Research and Professional Experience:

Position	University/Institution
Associate Professor II	Institute of Advanced Study in Science & Technology (IASST), Guwahati, Assam
Associate Professor I	Institute of Advanced Study in Science & Technology (IASST), Guwahati, Assam
Assistant Professor II	IASST, Guwahati, Assam
Biotechnologist & Plant Breeder	Tocklai Tea Research Institute, TRA, Jorhat, Assam & North Bengal Regional R&D Centre, (TRA), West Bengal
Project PI, SERC Young Scientist Project, DST, Govt. of India	Biotechnology Div. NEIST (CSIR), Jorhat, Assam
Research Associate	IMTECH (CSIR), Chandigarh
Senior Research Fellow (CSIR)	Biotechnology Div. NEIST (CSIR), Jorhat, Assam
LTM Fellowship (Mumbai)	Biotechnology Div. NEIST (CSIR), Jorhat, Assam
Project Assistant	Biotechnology Div. NEIST (CSIR), Jorhat, Assam

Professional Appointments: Associate Professor II, Life Sciences Division, Microbial Biotechnology Laboratory, Institute of Advanced Study in Science & Technology (IASST), Guwahati, Assam

Honors: Botany, Specialization in Microbiology

Publications from the Last 3 Years

1. Majumdar, Sristi, Debajit Thakur, and Devasish Chowdhury. "DNA carbon-nanodots based electrochemical biosensor for detection of mutagenic nitrosamines." *ACS Applied Bio Materials* 3, no. 3 (2020): 1796-1803.
2. Borah, Atlanta, and Debajit Thakur. "Phylogenetic and functional characterization of culturable endophytic actinobacteria associated with Camellia spp. for growth promotion in commercial tea cultivars." *Frontiers in Microbiology* 11 (2020): 318.
3. Dutta, Jintu, and Debajit Thakur. "Evaluation of antagonistic and plant growth promoting potential of Streptomyces sp. TT3 isolated from tea (Camellia sinensis) rhizosphere soil." *Current Microbiology* 77, no. 8 (2020): 1829-1838.
4. Hazarika, Shabiha Nudrat, and Debajit Thakur. "Actinobacteria." In *Beneficial Microbes in Agro-Ecology*, pp. 443-476. Academic Press, 2020.
5. Barman, Ananya, Archana Nath, and Debajit Thakur. "Identification and characterization of fungi associated with blister blight lesions of tea (Camellia sinensis L. Kuntze) isolated from Meghalaya, India." *Microbiological Research* 240 (2020): 126561.
6. Chowdhury, Devasish, Sristi Majumdar, and Debajit Thakur. "Actinobacteria mediated synthesis of bio-conjugate of carbon dot with enhanced biological activity." *Applied Nanoscience* 10, no. 7 (2020): 2199-2206.
7. Dutta, Jintu, and Debajit Thakur. "Diversity of culturable bacteria endowed with antifungal metabolites biosynthetic characteristics associated with tea rhizosphere soil of Assam, India." *BMC Microbiology* 21, no. 1 (2021): 1-13.
8. Bhattacharya, Anupam, Simang Champramary, Tanya Tripathi, Debajit Thakur, Ilya Ioshikhes, Satyendra Kumar Singh, and Soumyadeep Nandi. "Identification of the conserved long non-coding RNAs in myogenesis." *BMC Genomics* 22, no. 1 (2021): 1-19.
9. Konwar, Aditya Narayan, Shabiha Nudrat Hazarika, Pranami Bharadwaj, and Debajit Thakur. "Emerging Non-Traditional Approaches to Combat Antibiotic Resistance." *Current Microbiology* 79, no. 11 (2022): 1-15.

10. Kashyap, Bhaswati, Kangkon Saikia, Suman Kumar Samanta, Debajit Thakur, Sanjay Kumar Banerjee, Jagat Chandra Borah, and Narayan Chandra Talukdar. "Kaempferol 3-O-rutinoside from Antidesma acidum Retz. Stimulates glucose uptake through SIRT1 induction followed by GLUT4 translocation in skeletal muscle L6 cells." *Journal of Ethnopharmacology* 301 (2023): 115788.
11. Borah, Atlanta, Shabiha Nudrat Hazarika, and Debajit Thakur. "Potentiality of actinobacteria to combat against biotic and abiotic stresses in tea [Camellia sinensis (L) O. Kuntze]." *Journal of Applied Microbiology* 133, no. 4 (2022): 2314-2330.
12. Thakur, Debajit, Ananya Barman, and Manash Jyoti Deka. "*In vitro* antagonistic efficacy of a Paenibacillus sp. BTA27 against tea blister blight associated fungal pathogens." (2022).
13. Mazumdar, Rajkumari, and Debajit Thakur. "Therapeutic Applications of Nanotechnology in the Prevention of Infectious Diseases." In *Emerging Nanomaterials for Advanced Technologies*, pp. 323-343. Springer, Cham, 2022.
14. Das, Rictika, and Debajit Thakur. "Recent Developments in Nanotechnological Interventions for Pesticide Remediation." *Emerging Nanomaterials for Advanced Technologies* (2022): 553-580.
15. Hazarika, Shabiha Nudrat, Pranami Bharadwaj, Aditya Narayan Konwar, and Debajit Thakur. "Cloning and Heterologous Expression of Natural Products from Actinobacteria." In *Actinobacteria*, pp. 135-161. Springer, Singapore, 2022.
16. Hazarika, Shabiha Nudrat, Kangkon Saikia, and Debajit Thakur. "Characterization and selection of endophytic actinobacteria derived from commercial Tea plant grown in Northeast India for growth and disease management in host and non-host plants." *Frontiers in Plant Science* (2022): 4573.
17. Saikia, Juri, Rajkumari Mazumdar, and Debajit Thakur. "Phylogenetic Affiliation of Endophytic Actinobacteria Associated with Selected Orchid Species and Their Role in Growth Promotion and Suppression of Phytopathogens." *Frontiers in Plant Science* (2022): 4746.
18. Mazumdar, Rajkumari, Partha Pratim Dutta, Juri Saikia, Jagat Chandra Borah and Debajit Thakur. "Streptomyces sp. PBR11, a forest-derived soil actinomycetia with antimicrobial potentials." *Microbiology Spectrum* (2022) (accepted)

Juri Saikia

Affiliation: Institute of Advanced Study in Science and Technology (IASST), Gauhati University

Education: Master's in Biotechnology
Date of PhD Registration: 06-03-2017
Name of Supervisor: Dr. Debajit Thakur
Registration: BT-04/16

Institutional Address: Institute of Advanced Study in Science and Technology, Garchuk, Paschim Boragaon, Vigyan Path, Guwahati- 781035, Assam, India

Research Experience: Title: "Phylogenetic and functional characterization of endophytic bacterial community prevalent in different orchid species of Assam and their role in growth promotion and disease suppression."
Award: Rajiv Gandhi National Fellow
Funding agency: UGC (University Grant Commission)
Duration: 5 Years

Honors: Biotechnology

Publications from the Last 3 Years

1. Saikia, Juri, Rajkumari Mazumdar, and Debajit Thakur. "Phylogenetic Affiliation of Endophytic Actinobacteria Associated with Selected Orchid Species and Their Role in Growth Promotion and Suppression of Phytopathogens." *Frontiers in Plant Science* (2022): 4746.
2. Mazumdar, Rajkumari, Partha Pratim Dutta, Juri Saikia, Jagat Chandra Borah and Debajit Thakur. "Streptomyces sp. PBR11, a forest-derived soil actinomycetia with antimicrobial potentials. " *Microbiology Spectrum* (2022) (accepted)

Rajkumari Mazumdar

Affiliation: Institute of Advanced Study in Science and Technology (IASST), Cotton University

Education: Master's in Biotechnology
Date of PhD Registration: 06-02-2019
Name of Supervisor: Dr. Debajit Thakur
Registration: MBB1891009

Institutional Address: Institute of Advanced Study in Science and Technology, Garchuk, Paschim Boragaon, Vigyan Path, Guwahati- 781035, Assam, India

Research Experience:

- One year project entitled "Assessment of the acquisition of drug resistant urinary tract infection (UTI) pathogens infect woman in Guwahati city, Assam and in-vitro evaluation of microbial secondary metabolites against drug resistant UTI pathogens" under internship mode of DST-KIRAN WOS-B (Women scientist - B)
- Title: "Exploration and conservation of microbial resources prevalent in protected forest ecosystems and tea rhizosphere soil of Assam."
  Sanction No. BT/PR12956/NDB/39/504/2015;
  Sanction date: 27-02-2017
  Funding Agency: DBT, Govt. of India
  Duration: 3 years.
  Involved as: Project Technical Assistant

Honors: Biotechnology

Publications from the Last 3 Years:

1. Mazumdar, Rajkumari, and Debajit Thakur. "Therapeutic Applications of Nanotechnology in the Prevention of Infectious Diseases." In *Emerging Nanomaterials for Advanced Technologies*, pp. 323-343. Springer, Cham, 2022.
2. Saikia, Juri, Rajkumari Mazumdar, and Debajit Thakur. "Phylogenetic Affiliation of Endophytic Actinobacteria Associated with Selected Orchid Species and Their Role in Growth Promotion and Suppression of Phytopathogens." *Frontiers in Plant Science* (2022): 4746.

3. Mazumdar, Rajkumari, Partha Pratim Dutta, Juri Saikia, Jagat Chandra Borah and Debajit Thakur. "Streptomyces sp. PBR11, a forest-derived soil actinomycetia with antimicrobial potentials. " *Microbiology Spectrum* (2022) (accepted)

Chapter 4

Infectious Diseases: Antibiotic Resistance and Stewardship

Rajkumari Mazumdar[1,2], Juri Saikia[1,3] and Debajit Thakur[1,*]

[1] Microbial Biotechnology Laboratory, Life Sciences Division, Institute of Advanced Study in Science and Technology (IASST), Guwahati, India
[2] Department of Molecular Biology and Biotechnology, Cotton University, Guwahati, India
[3] Department of Biotechnology, Gauhati University, Guwahati, India

Abstract

Infectious diseases are illnesses caused by pathogenic microorganisms that enter our bodies from the outside. They can sometimes be caught by other people, the environment, animal contact, or insect bites. Some infections are so mild that we might not notice any symptoms, while others can be fatal. Existing and emerging infectious diseases pose significant challenges to public health outcomes around the globe. Pathogenic bacteria continue to be a severe health concern, causing many fatalities and hospitalizations yearly. Due to the development of new variants of drug-resistant pathogenic microorganisms, the treatment and immunization of infectious diseases have become even more challenging in recent years. Existing diagnostic techniques are inefficient because they lack speed and ultra-sensitivity. Therefore, novel therapeutic and diagnostic approaches are required.

[*] Corresponding Author's Email: debajitthakur@yahoo.co.uk.

In: Infectious Diseases
Editor: Yvette S. Brewer
ISBN: 979-8-88697-657-1

The primary goal of this study is to highlight current trends in antibiotic resistance as well as novel therapeutic prospects for future disease management and control advancements.

Keywords: infectious diseases, antimicrobial resistance, pathogenic bacteria, WHO, actinobacteria, antimicrobial peptides, nanoparticle

Introduction

Infectious diseases are caused by pathogenic microorganisms that enter our bodies from the outside. Pathogenic bacteria remain a major public health concern, resulting in numerous deaths and hospitalizations every year. Bacteria are single-cell microscopic organisms (microbes) that exist everywhere, including inside our bodies and on our skin. They are necessary for sustaining the ecosystem in which we live. The majority of bacteria in the environment do not cause infection. Many bacteria are harmless or even beneficial, but some are infective and produce toxins that cause infections and the public's health is significantly impacted by these bacterial infections [1]. Bacterial infection can infect any part of the human body. Each bacterial species prefers to infect definite organs over others. *Neisseria meningitidis*, for example, mainly infects the meninges of the central nervous system, resulting in meningitis, but it can also infect the lungs, resulting in pneumonia. However, it is not a source of skin infection. Individuals commonly carry *Staphylococcus aureus* on their skin or mucous membranes, which frequently causes soft tissue and skin infections. But it can also spread easily all over the body through the bloodstream and can infect the lungs, abdomen, heart valves, and nearly any other site. The bacterium *Mycobacterium tuberculosis* (MT) is the cause of the contagious disease recognized as tuberculosis (TB) [2]. It typically migrates to the lungs after entering the body through the nose [3]. In contrast, *Salmonella* enters the mouth (via contaminated food or water) and travels to the gut lining, where it affects the intestinal tract [4].

Antibiotics are medications used to treat or prevent bacterial infections. They kill bacteria or make it difficult for bacteria to grow and multiply. However, the issue of bacterial resistance to antibiotics is one that is rapidly growing and may have extremely negative effects. Resistance among bacterial pathogens has been recognized as a major public health threat affecting humans globally. The discovery and commercialization of antimicrobial drugs to treat various infections transformed modern medicine and changed the therapeutic framework. Antibiotics have undoubtedly become one of the most important medical interventions required for the development of complex medical approaches such as advanced surgical procedures, organ transplantation, and cancer treatment [6]. Unfortunately, the rapid rise in antibiotic resistance among common bacterial pathogens is now risking this therapeutic breakthrough, threatening the successful outcomes of critically ill patients. In fact, the World Health Organization (WHO) has classified antibiotic resistance as one of the top three public health threats of the twenty-first century [7]. Understanding the true burden of resistance is a major challenge in combating antibiotic resistance, especially in areas where surveillance is limited, and data is scarce. The WHO nevertheless regularly publishes data and information on the burden of infectious diseases in order to notify the public, policy-makers, and healthcare professionals about the most significant illnesses in terms of morbidity and mortality [8].

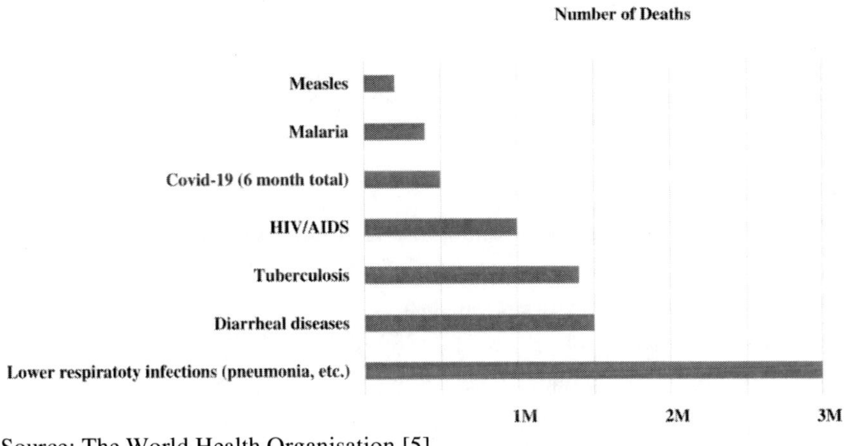

Source: The World Health Organisation [5].

Figure 1. Annual deaths from each infectious diseases (from 2015-2020).

Healthcare-Associated Infections

The terms "hospital-acquired infections" (HAI) or "healthcare-associated infections" (HCAI) refer to nosocomial acquired infections that develop while receiving treatment at a hospital or from a healthcare practitioner [9]. Usually, these infections develop after being hospitalized and become apparent 48 hours after being admitted. Central line-associated bloodstream infections, hospital-acquired pneumonia, catheter-associated urinary tract infections (UTIs), surgical site infections, ventilator-associated pneumonia, and *Clostridium difficile* infections are cases of HCAIs [10]. Approximately 7% of patients in developed countries and 10% in underdeveloped nations will develop at least one HAI. Additionally, these illnesses place a heavy financial strain on society. However, a significant portion can be prevented by active infection prevention and control (IPC) management. A thorough review by WHO in 2011 revealed an incredibly fragmented image of the endemic burden of HCAI in poor nations [11]. Only limited evidence regarding HCAI was available from some places, while many countries had no data (66%). Much research conducted in low-resource healthcare settings found HCAI rates greater than in developed nations. In hospitals, the prevalence of HCAI ranged from 5.7% to 19.1%, with a total frequency of 10%. Surgical Site Infection (SSI) is the most common type of infection in low- and middle-income countries (LIMICs), with incidence rates varying from 1.2 to 23.6% per 100 surgical procedures and a total frequency of 11.8%. SSI rates in developed countries range from 1.2% to 5.2%. Intensive care units (ICUs) have a higher risk of HCAI, with about 30% of patients having at least one episode with significant morbidity and mortality.

According to a recent WHO report (6 May 2022), out of 100 patients, 7 patients in high-income countries and 15 patients in LIMICs will contract at least one HAI during their hospital stay [12]. On average, one in every ten affected patients would die as a result of HAI. People in intensive care and infants are particularly at risk. According to the report, one in every four hospital-treated sepsis cases and approximately half of all sepsis with organ failure treated in adult intensive-care units are health-care-related [11, 13].

The most important strategies and perspectives for improving HCAI surveillance and control are:

1. Local factors of the HCAI burden must be identified.
2. National processes for reporting and surveillance should be improved.
3. Making sure that the fundamental elements of infection control are in place on a national and hospital level.
4. Precautionary measures are being implemented, mainly best hand hygiene practices at the bedside.
5. Increasing employee awareness and responsibility.

6. Ensure that the institutional level has the bare minimum of infrastructure and dedicated resources for HCAI surveillance, including the capacity of microbial laboratories.
7. Investigating the role of patients and their families in the reporting and management of HCAI.

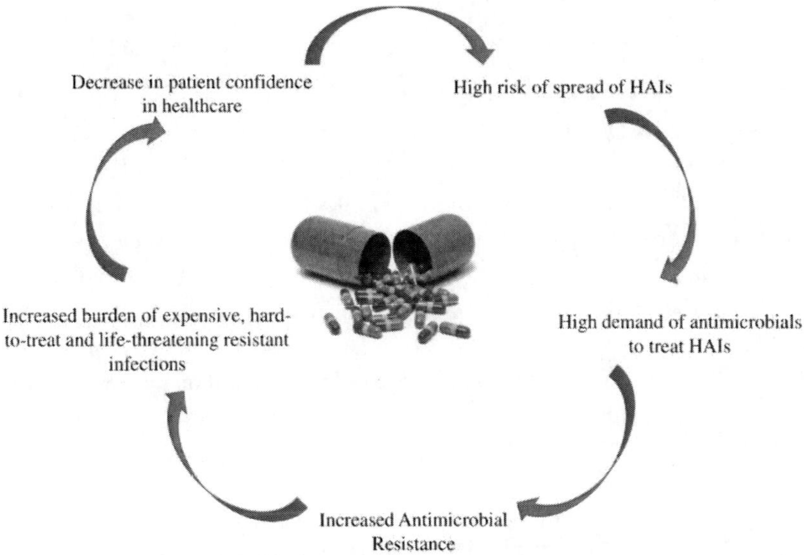

Figure 2. Factors responsible for healthcare-associated infections (HCAI).

Infection Prevention and Control (IPC)

IPC is a pragmatic, evidence-based strategy that protect patients and healthcare professionals from avoidable infections. Impactful IPC necessitates continuous action at all levels of the health system, including decision makers, facility managers, health workers, and those who access health care services. It is not possible to achieve quality healthcare delivery without effective IPC. Programs to facilitate IPC are extremely crucial in low- and middle-income countries, where secondary infections can have a negative impact on healthcare conditions and medical hygiene standards [12]. No health authority can afford to ignore the ongoing issue of HAIs. To aid in this effort, WHO has developed a number of initiatives that promote evidence-based recommendations and operational procedures and reduce the spread of preventable infections. The first WHO Global Patient Challenge laid the groundwork for the IPC Global Unit, which works to help countries build capacity for IPC action. Through this program, WHO offers technical support for establishing national IPC policies and guidelines, organizes meetings centered on developing guidelines, and offers ongoing assistance to healthcare professional [14].

Strategies for the Prevention and Control of Health-Care Acquired Infection

Carbapenem-resistant *Acinetobacter baumannii* (CRAB), carbapenem-resistant Enterobacteriaceae (CRE), and carbapenem-resistant *Pseudomonas aeruginosa* (CRPsA) are carbapenem-resistant gram-negative bacteria that pose a serious threat to public health and are responsible for most of the healthcare-acquired infections [15, 16]. The World Health Organization has designated CRE-CRAB-CRPsA prevention and control as an urgent priority for the global health agenda. The first global guidelines for the prevention and control of CRE-CRAB-CRPsA in healthcare facilities were established on October 14, 2017 [15].

They are planned to provide scientific proof-based guidance on early detection and measures required to properly prevent CRE-CRAB-CRPsA colonization and/or infection in acute health care settings. They serve as a foundation for developing and/or strengthening national IPC policies and programs to control CRE-CRAB-CRPsA transmission in various healthcare institutions and centers. These guidelines build on the broad standards established by the World Health Organization Publication Guidelines on core elements of infection prevention and control management programs at the national and acute healthcare facility levels. According to the WHO, effective IPC programs can cut healthcare-associated infections by 70% [14].

Antibiotic Resistance

In 1928, British scientist Alexander Fleming discovered a compound that could killed *Staphylococcus aureus*. He called this compound penicillin, named after the *Penicillium* mold that made it. With the discovery of penicillin and the advent of the antibiotic era, the body's defences gained a strong ally.

Penicillin's success sparked a race to develop new antibiotics [17]. The development of antibiotics changed the course of human history by making previously incurable diseases treatable and enabling the safe completion of medical procedures like surgery and chemotherapy. The wellbeing has significantly improved, and millions of lives have been saved. Antibiotics have proven to be extremely effective. However, at the same time, optimism over them has been dampened by a phenomenon known as antibiotic resistance. Antibiotics have been used so extensively that many of them have lost their ability to combat bacteria. Overuse of antibiotics has resulted in the emergence of drug-resistant pathogens. Antibiotic-resistant bacterial strains are already caused 4·95 million deaths in 2019 and this number is anticipated to rise exponentially in the absence of immediate action [18].

Antibiotics changed our world by allowing previously incurable diseases to be treated and medical treatments like surgery and chemotherapy to be conducted safely. Our standard of living has significantly increased, and millions of lives have been saved [19]. But our time with these drugs is coming to an end. Despite the availability of new antibiotics, the rate of development of new drugs has lagged behind the rate of resistance. Usually, the more often antibiotics are used, the more bacteria adapt and find new ways to survive, which means they become resistant to antibiotics. The misuse of antibiotics and inadequate infection prevention and control, are the main causes of antibiotic resistance [20]. Antibiotic resistance presents a severe threat to global health and is expected to have a considerable impact on both health and the economy, particularly in LMICs. [21]. Drug-resistant bacterial infections (including tuberculosis) are expected to kill at least 700,000 people worldwide each year, with 90% of these deaths occurring in LMICs such as Africa and Asia [21, 22]. According to the World Bank, drug-resistant illnesses would cost the globe up to 3.8 percentage of its yearly gross domestic product (GDP) by the year 2050 [23].

How Does Antibiotic Resistance Develop?

Antibiotic resistance in bacteria can emerge in a number of ways [24]:

1. Some bacteria can modify their outer membrane, making it impossible for the antibiotic to bind to the bacterium it is meant to kill.

2. Some bacteria have the ability to "neutralize" an antibiotic by modifying it in a way that renders it useless.
3. Some bacteria have pumping mechanisms that allow antibiotics to leave their bodies before they become active.
4. Bacteria can also develop resistance by altering their genetic material. Bacteria can sometimes survive after being exposed to drugs by developing a resistance to the antibiotic. If even one microbe develops resistance to an antibiotic, it has the potential to reproduce and replace all of the bacteria that were killed.

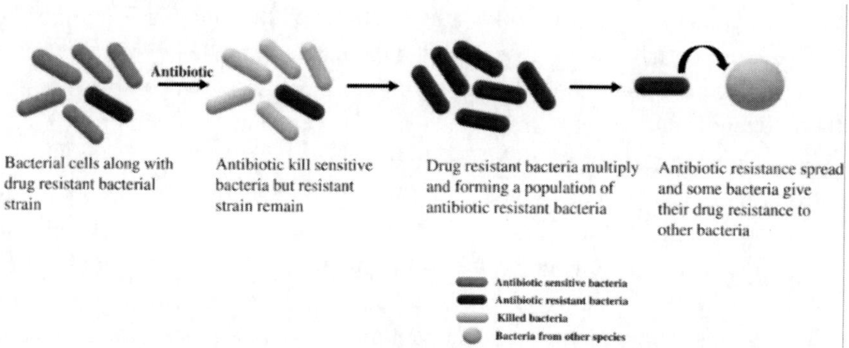

Figure 3. A schematic representation showing how a bacterial population can develop antibiotic resistance; Bacterial growth is inhibited or killed by antibiotics. However, a limited percentage of bacteria develop antibiotic resistance naturally. Repeated exposure to various antibiotics causes susceptible bacteria to perish, allowing drug-resistant bacteria to thrive [25]. It indicates that some pathogenic bacteria become more adept at resisting antibiotics and develop antibiotic-resistant strains. The remaining drug-resistant bacteria can then thrive and even transmit their drug-resistant traits to other bacteria through a process known as horizontal gene transfer (HGT) [26].

The (WHO) has identified 12 families of drug-resistant bacteria that pose the biggest threat to human health and necessitating the urgent need for novel drug therapies to combat drug resistance. Three bacteria have been identified as top priorities for new treatments by the WHO [27]. They are:

- *Acinetobacter baumannii*: Resistant to a class of antibiotics known as carbapenems and can cause many types of infections in hospitalized patients, such as pneumonia, wound and blood infections.

- *Pseudomonas aeruginosa*: Resistant to carbapenems and are responsible for lung infections, burn wound infection and severe blood infections.
- Enterobacterales is an order of gram-negative bacteria inhabits the intestines of animals and are resistant to carbapenems and extended-spectrum cephalosporins. They spread easily and are the major cause of urinary tract infections (UTIs) and bloodstream infections in hospitalized patients.

Table 1. List of drug resistant bacterial strains identified by WHO

High priority	
Neisseria gonorrhoeae	Cephalosporin-resistant, fluoroquinolone-resistant
Salmonellae	Fluoroquinolone-resistant
Enterococcus faecium	Vancomycin-resistant
Staphylococcus aureus	Methicillin-resistant, vancomycin-intermediate and resistant
Helicobacter pylori	Clarithromycin-resistant
Campylobacter sp.	Fluoroquinolone-resistant
Medium priority	
Streptococcus pneumoniae	Penicillin-non-susceptible
Campylobacter sp.	Fluoroquinolone-resistant
Shigella sp.	Fluoroquinolone-resistant

WHO Response on Antibiotic Resistance

WHO prioritizes the fight against antibiotic resistance. In May 2015, the World Health Assembly approved a global action plan on antimicrobial resistance, including antibiotic resistance. The global action plan aims to provide medications that are both safe and effective for the prevention and treatment of various infectious diseases [28].

The "Global action plan on antimicrobial resistance" has five strategic goals:

1. To raise awareness and conception of antimicrobial resistance.
2. To improve research and surveillance on antimicrobial resistance.
3. To decrease the likelihood of infection.
4. To improve the use of antimicrobial medications.
5. To ensure sustainable investment in combating antimicrobial resistance.

Heads of State endorsed a political declaration at the UN General Assembly in New York in September 2016 that showed the world's commitment to implementing a detailed and coordinated strategy to address antimicrobial resistance across various sectors, particularly in all health sectors. The WHO is assisting Member states in establishing national action plans on antibiotic resistance based on the global action plan [29].

Antimicrobial Resistance Surveillance (ARS)

Surveillance is a crucial tool for gathering information that supports standardized methods for collecting, analyzing and sharing data on antimicrobial resistance at a global level [30, 31]. ARS programs can be categorized into two main groups according to their primary goals: (1) public health ARS programs and (2) industry-sponsored/product-oriented ARS programs. Public health ARS programs primarily concentrate on health care and infection control, while industry ARS programs typically focus on an investigational or recently approved molecule/s [30, 32]. Surveillance is a crucial tool for informing policy and infection prevention and control strategies. Importantly, it is the cornerstone for assessing the spread of AMR and to inform and monitor the impact of local, national and global strategies.

On October 22, 2015, WHO launched the Global Antimicrobial Resistance and Use Surveillance System (GLASS), the first global collaborative effort to standardize AMR surveillance [32, 33]. GLASS was established to assist the second goal of the GAP-AMR initiative, "strengthen knowledge through surveillance and research," and to continue filling knowledge gaps with the aim of informing strategies at all levels. This goal was endorsed by the 68th World Health Assembly in resolution WHA68.7. GLASS provides a standardized approach to the collection, analysis, interpretation and sharing of data by countries and seeks to actively support capacity building and monitor the status of existing and new national surveillance systems [33]. Furthermore, GLASS promotes a shift from surveillance approaches based solely on laboratory data that includes epidemiological, clinical, and population-level information. GLASS has been conceived to progressively incorporate data from surveillance of AMR in humans, such as monitoring of resistance and the use of antimicrobial medicines, including AMR in the food chain and in the environment [33, 34]. GLASS is supported by the WHO AMR Surveillance and Quality Assessment Collaborating Centers Network and operates at all three levels of WHO:

headquarters, regional and country offices. It has a full dedication from participating countries and collaborates with AMR regional networks such as the Central Asian and European Surveillance of Antimicrobial Resistance (CAESAR), the European Antimicrobial Resistance Surveillance Network (EARS-Net), the Latin American Network for Antimicrobial Resistance Surveillance, and the Western Pacific Regional Antimicrobial Consumption Surveillance System WPRACSS [33].

Antimicrobial Stewardship (AMS)

Stewardship is defined as "the thoughtful and accountable management of anything entrusted to one's care"[35]. It was first utilized in the healthcare setting as a strategy for optimizing antibiotic consumption, which was termed as "Antimicrobial Stewardship" (AMS) [36]. Since then, stewardship has been used in the perspective of governance of the health sector as a whole, taking ownership of the population's health and wellbeing and guiding healthcare systems at the national and international levels. Additionally, it encourages the appropriate use antibiotics and other antimicrobial agents, enhances patient outcomes, lowers microbial resistance and HCAI, saves healthcare costs amongst others and reduces the spread of infections caused by MDR pathogens [37, 38]. National action plans have also been implemented by nations like India, China, South Africa, Kenya, Argentina, Uruguay, Malaysia, and Colombia to enhance antibiotic stewardship and reduce AMR [39].

Objectives of an AMS Programme

1. To optimize and improve antibiotic use.
2. To encourage a change in how people prescribe and dispense antibiotics.
3. To enhance the quality of care and improve patient outcomes.
4. To save money on unnecessary healthcare expenses.
5. To reduce further emergence, selection and spread of AMR.
6. To extend the life of existing antibiotics.
7. To reduce the negative effects of AMR on the economy.
8. To increase the ability of healthcare professionals to use finest practices when it comes to the prudent use of antibiotics.

According to ReAct Report, 2021 [40], two main actions are required to keep up with the rapidly increasing antibiotic resistance:

1. The effectiveness of currently available antibiotics must be maintained, in part through infection prevention methods and by optimizing their use through stewardship.
2. To enable the development of novel and efficient types of antibiotics and the antibiotic pipeline needs to be replenished regularly.

Search for New Antibacterial Agents to Combat Antibiotic Resistance

The golden age of natural product antibiotic research began with the discovery of penicillin in 1928 and peaked in the middle of the 1950s [6, 38]. The discovery of new antibiotics has gradually declined and majority of pharmaceutical firms are no longer engaged in this endeavor. Half of the antibiotics currently in use were developed in the 1950s. Since then, antibiotic discovery and development have become more difficult, complex and expensive [41]. To slow the emergence and spread of resistance, new antibiotics are urgently needed with short treatment durations and limitations on their use. Even when new antibiotics are developed, they hardly target the drug-resistant bacteria and are only approved for use in handful of countries. Between 1999 and 2014, only 12 of the 25 new antibiotics that were released on the market received approval in more than ten countries [42].

The battle between both antibiotics and antibiotic-resistant bacteria keeps going. The more scientists develop novel and efficient antibiotics, the more frequently bacteria will change their genetic mutations and adjust their defences mechanism. To address the issue of antimicrobial resistance, novel drugs must be discovered, which is a critical component of a coordinated antimicrobial resistance response [43]. Antibiotic resistance is a global health and economic problem, prompting researchers to look for new antibacterial agents to combat resistant bacterial strains that increase mortality and epidemics. According to a WHO report, lack of private investment and failure to produce novel antibiotics made it more difficult to fight against drug-resistant infections [44]. As a result, there is an urgent need for novel strategies and resources that can address the problems of AMR.

Actinobacteria: Prolific Producer of Antibiotics

Drug-resistant bacterial strains are developing more rapidly than new antibiotics. Many scientists and pharmaceutical firms have been working hard to isolate and screen actinobacteria from various habitats in order to develop new antibiotics [45, 46]. Nearly 80% of the world antibiotics used today are produced by actinobacteria, primarily from the genera *Streptomyces* and *Micromonospora* [47]. They are the main producers of natural products and have a long history of producing effective antimicrobials agents with potential pharmaceutical properties such astetracycline, ivermectin, streptomycin, and nystatin [48]. They are well-known for producing structurally diverged group of bioactive secondary metabolites. These bioactive compounds have distinct chemical assemblages that may help in the catalysis or synthesis of novel antimicrobial drugs effective against a wide range of drug-resistant pathogens.[49].

The most important antibiotics produced in nature by Actinobacteria are summarized in Table 1A, 1B, 1C, 1D [19].

Table 1A. Natural β-lactam antibiotics and β-lactamase inhibitors produced by Actinobacteria

β-Lactams		Producer Microorganism
Penicillin	Penicillin N	*S. lipmanii*; *S. microflavus*; *S. griseus* subsp. *Cryophilus*; *S. cattleya*
Cephalosporines	Cephamycins	*S. clavuligerus*; *S. griseus*; *S. lactamdurans*; *S. chartreusis*; *S. cinnamonensis*; *S. fimbriatus*; *S. halstedii*; *S. rochei*; *S. viridochromogenes*; *S. wadayamensis*; *S. Jumonjineneis*; *S. lipmanii*; *S. panayaensis*; *Amycolatopsis lactamdurans*; *S. cattleya; S. heteromorphus*
	Cephalosporines	*S. microflavus*; *S. lipmanii*; *S. clavuligerus*; *S. hygroscopicus*
Carbapenems	Thienamycins	*S. cattleya*; *S. griseus* subsp. *Cryophilus*; *S. penemifaciens*; *S. flavogriseus*; *S. olivaceus*; *S. cremeus* subsp. *auratilis*; *S. flavoviridis*
Monobactam	Nocardicins	*Nocardia uniformis*; *Nocardia uniformis* subsp. *Tsuyamanensis*; *Streptomyces alcalophilus* sp. nov.; *Actinosynnema mirum*; *Microtetraspora caesia*
PBP inhibitors	Clavulanic acid	*S. clavuligerus*; *S. jumonjinesis*; *S. katsuharamanus*
	Olivanic acid	*S. olivaceus; S. griseus* subsp. *cryophilus*

Table 1B. Natural tetracycline antibiotics produced by Actinobacteria

Tetracycline Antibiotics	Producer Microorganism
Tetracycline	*S. aureofaciens*; *S. avellaneus*; *S. lusitanus*; *S. viridifaciens*
Chlortetracycline	*S. lusitanus*; *S. aureofaciens*; *S. lividans*
Oxytetracycline	*S. alboflavus*; *Streptomyces albofaciens*; *Streptomyces erumpens*; *S. griseus*; *S. platensis*; *S. rimosus* subsp. *rimosus*; *S. varsoviensis*
6-demethyltetracycline	*S. aureofaciens*

Table 1C. Natural aminoglycoside antibiotics produced by Actinobacteria

Aminoglycoside Antibiotics	Producer Microorganism
Streptomycin	*S. griseus; S. bikiniensis; S. streptomycinii; S. ornatus; S. humidus; S. subrutilus; S. mashuensis; S. glaucescens; S. griseocarneus; Streptomyces rimosus subsp. rimosus; S. galbus*
Neomycin	*S. fradiae; S. catenulae; S. chrestomyceticus; S. albogriseolus*
Tobramycin	*Streptoalloteichus hindustanus; S. tenebrarius; S. cremeus*
Kanamycin	*Streptoalloteichus hindustanus; S. tenebrarius; S. cremeus*
Paromomycym	*S. rimosus var. paromomycinus; S. catenulae; S. chrestomyceticus; S. rimosus; S. fradiae*
Gentamycin	*Micromonospora purpurea; Micromonospora pallida; Micromonospora echinospora*

Table 1D. Natural peptide antibiotics produced by Actinobacteria

Peptide Antibiotics		Producer Microorganism
Glycopeptides	vancomycin	*Amycolatopsis orientalis* subsp. *Orientalis*
Lipopeptides	daptomycin	*Streptomyces sp.* KCTC12267BP; *S. roseosporus*
Streptogramins	Streptogramins A and B	*S. halstedii*; *S. pristinaespiralis*; *S. virginiae*

S: Streptomyces sp.

Antimicrobial Peptides

Antimicrobial peptides (AMPs), also known as host defence peptides (HDPs), are a family of short peptides that are abundant in nature and play a vital role in the innate immune systems of various organisms [50]. The occurrence of antibiotic-resistant microbes, as well as growing concerns about the use of antimicrobial drugs, led to the development of AMPs, which have a promising future in the pharmaceutical sectors. Different types of synthetic AMPs have been developed in laboratories and some are naturally present in animals and plants. However, they are also produced by microbes (bacteria and yeast) [51]. AMPs exhibited diverse bioactivities, such as antimicrobial and anti-mitogenic agents, as well as an anticancer, anti-inflammatory, and immunological modulator. AMPs represent a potential replacement for a wide range of regularly prescribed medications. Additionally, many research suggest that AMPs have significant therapeutic effect in both *in vitro* and *in vivo* studies [52]. AMPs, nanoparticles (NPs), as well as the development of combinatorial treatments, are the most novel approaches for combating infectious diseases caused by XDR (Extensively drug-resistant) and MDR (Multidrug-resistant) bacteria [53].

In order to combat various infectious organisms, mostly MDR bacteria, the use of AMPs, either alone or in conjunction with standard drugs has shown to be successful [54]. Recent investigations have demonstrated that AMPs and antibiotics work together synergistically. Akbari and his co-workers (2019) reported the synergistic effects between melittin, a cationic amphipathic peptide, and antibiotics such doripenem, colistin, doxycycline, and ceftazidime against MDR isolates of *Acinetobacter baumannii* and *Pseudomonas aeruginosa* [55]. Various natural and synthesized AMPs, such as nisin, cecropins, and defensins, have demonstrated strong antibacterial action against both gram-positive and gram-negative bacteria. According to recent findings, AMPs P5 (YIRKIRRFFKKLKKILKK-NH2) and P9 (SYERKINRHFKTLKKNLKKK-NH2) which are designed based on Aristicluthys nobilia interferon-I inhibit MRSA with low cytotoxicity [56].

Nanomaterials: Role in Overcoming Antibiotic Resistance

The growing concern about multi-drug resistant bacterial strains and biofilm-related infections drives the demand for new bactericidal agents. As an alternative to antibiotics, nanoparticles (NPs) are increasingly being employed to target pathogenic bacteria [57]. As a result, new and emerging nanoparticle-based materials have received considerable attention in the field of antimicrobial chemotherapy [58]. The delivery of drugs to the target at the appropriate doses and at the right times is the most crucial requirement for any effective therapeutic agent. Nanomaterials are one of the most promising smart drug delivery systems because of their exceptional size and surface features [59]. Nanomedicine plays a crucial role in increasing the efficacy of currently used therapeutics by enhancing the physicochemical properties and stability of antibiotics, and the prolongation of controlled drug release, as well as enabling targeted drug delivery to the site of infection [60]. Another interesting characteristic of nanomaterials is their antibacterial properties. They are widely employed as an antibacterial agent to kill pathogenic and drug-resistant bacteria [59]. Particularly NPs have proven to provide broad-spectrum antibacterial effects against both Gram-positive and Gram-negative bacteria. For instance, Ag NPs exhibit concentration-dependent antibacterial action against *Escherichia coli* and *Pseudomonas aeruginosa*, and ZnO NPs showed antibacterial activity against *Staphylococcus aureus* [61].

Because they offer prolonged antimicrobial activity with negligible toxicity, nanomaterials are now a potential antimicrobial agent to control bacterial infections. This is in contrast to small molecular antimicrobial agents, which have transient activity and are toxic to the environment. The antimicrobial nanoparticle physically damages the cell membranes of the organism, blocking the growth of drug-resistant bacteria [62]. Nanoparticle-based treatment appears to be a very promising technique for combating antibiotic resistance. As a result, conjugating antibiotics with nanoparticles may boost inhibition while minimizing the likelihood of drug resistance [63]. To treat a diverse range of microbial infections, including drug-resistant tuberculosis, antimicrobial agents are being specifically incorporated into polymer-coated crystalline nanoparticles, composite hydrogel/glass particles, PLGA, liposomes, homogenized particulate suspensions, cationic, dendrimers, silver nanoparticles, and gold nanoparticles [64].

Conclusion

Infectious diseases are still a leading cause of death in the modern world despite significant improvements in our understanding of how pathogens cause disease and the development of therapeutic interventions to combat infection. Monitoring the spread of infectious diseases is critical for improving public health because it allows us to reduce risks and prevent further transmission. Untreatable infections are becoming more prevalent in clinical settings as a result of the emergence of multidrug resistant pathogens. Due to the emergence of antibiotic resistance, the therapeutic approaches for treating infections are becoming increasingly limited, which increases the morbidity and mortality related to infections. This bleak picture has been exacerbated by a lack of antibiotic research and development. Therefore, it has become essential to conduct research and develop novel antimicrobial agents to reduce antimicrobial resistance. The choice of the appropriate combination therapy is essential for the prevention of infectious diseases. Combinatorial treatment opens the door to the development of antimicrobial therapies with broad-spectrum antibacterial action. Furthermore, to develop cutting-edge tactics to address the global threat posed by resistance, a thorough understanding of the mechanisms by which bacteria develop antibiotic resistance is important. By enhancing the supervision of patients, the quality of data in global AMR surveillance, supporting Global action plan on antimicrobial resistance, construction of proper laboratory infrastructures are essential to addressing the significant and global burden of AMR. In order to improve health and wellness, it is extremely important that various scientific disciplines share their experience, knowledge, technologies, and expertise.

References

[1] Doron, S., and S. L. Gorbach. "Bacterial infections: overview." *International Encyclopedia of Public Health* (2008): 273.

[2] Barberis, Ilaria, Nicola Luigi Bragazzi, Lucia Galluzzo, and Mariano Martini. "The history of tuberculosis: from the first historical records to the isolation of Koch's bacillus." *Journal of Preventive Medicine and Hygiene* 58, no. 1 (2017): E9.

[3] Long, Richard, Maziar Divangahi, and Kevin Schwartzman. "Chapter 2: Transmission and pathogenesis of tuberculosis." *Canadian Journal of Respiratory, Critical Care, and Sleep Medicine* 6, no. sup1 (2022): 22-32.

[4] Barnett, Richard. "Case histories Typhoid fever." *Lancet* 388, no. 10059 (2016): 2467-2467.

[5] Organisation, W. H., https://www.vox.com/2020/6/17/21289483/coronavirus-covid-19-vaccine-vaccinations-measles-malaria-tuberculosis. 2020.

[6] Hutchings, Matthew I., Andrew W. Truman, and Barrie Wilkinson. "Antibiotics: past, present and future." *Current Opinion in Microbiology* 51 (2019): 72-80.

[7] Munita, Jose M., and Cesar A. Arias. "Mechanisms of antibiotic resistance." *Microbiology Spectrum* 4, no. 2 (2016): 4-2.

[8] World Health Organisation., *The Global Burden of Disease: 2004 update*. 2008.

[9] Murhekar, Manoj V., and CP Girish Kumar. "Health-care-associated infection surveillance in India." *The Lancet Global Health* 10, no. 9 (2022): e1222-e1223.

[10] Monegro, Alberto F., Vijayadershan Muppidi, and Hariharan Regunath. "Hospital acquired infections." In *StatPearls [Internet]*. StatPearls Publishing, 2020.

[11] World Health Organisation., *Report on the Burden of Endemic Health Care-Associated Infection Worldwide.* 2011.

[12] World Health Organisation., *Global Report on Infection Prevention and Control.* 2022.

[13] Markwart, Robby, Hiroki Saito, Thomas Harder, Sara Tomczyk, Alessandro Cassini, Carolin Fleischmann-Struzek, Felix Reichert, Tim Eckmanns, and Benedetta Allegranzi. "Epidemiology and burden of sepsis acquired in hospitals and intensive care units: a systematic review and meta-analysis." *Intensive Care Medicine* 46, no. 8 (2020): 1536-1551.

[14] Balakrishnan, Vijay Shankar. "WHO's first global infection prevention and control report." *The Lancet Infectious Diseases* 22, no. 8 (2022): 1122.

[15] Tomczyk, Sara, Veronica Zanichelli, M. Lindsay Grayson, Anthony Twyman, Mohamed Abbas, Daniela Pires, Benedetta Allegranzi, and Stephan Harbarth. "Control of carbapenem-resistant Enterobacteriaceae, Acinetobacter baumannii, and Pseudomonas aeruginosa in healthcare facilities: a systematic review and reanalysis of quasi-experimental studies." *Clinical Infectious Diseases* 68, no. 5 (2019): 873-884.

[16] Nguyen, M., and S. G. Joshi. "Carbapenem resistance in Acinetobacter baumannii, and their importance in hospital-acquired infections: a scientific review." *Journal of Applied Microbiology* 131, no. 6 (2021): 2715-2738.

[17] Fisher, Margaret C. *Immunizations & Infectious Diseases: An Informed Parent's Guide*. American Academy of Pediatrics, 2006.

[18] Murray, Christopher JL, Kevin Shunji Ikuta, Fablina Sharara, Lucien Swetschinski, Gisela Robles Aguilar, Authia Gray, Chieh Han, Catherine Bisignano, Puja Rao, Eve Wool, Sarah C Johnson et al. "Global burden of bacterial antimicrobial resistance in 2019: a systematic analysis." *The Lancet* 399, no. 10325 (2022): 629-655.

[19] De Simeis, Davide, and Stefano Serra. "Actinomycetes: A never-ending source of bioactive compounds—An overview on antibiotics production." *Antibiotics* 10, no. 5 (2021): 483.

[20] Sartelli, M., C. Hardcastle, T., Catena, F., Chichom-Mefire, A., Coccolini, F., Dhingra, S., Haque, M., Hodonou, A., Iskandar, K., Labricciosa, F. M., Marmorale, C., Sall, I., & Pagani, L. "Antibiotic use in low and middle-income countries and the challenges of antimicrobial resistance in surgery." *Antibiotics* 9, no. 8 (2020): 497.

[21] Gandra, Sumanth, Gerardo Alvarez-Uria, Paul Turner, Jyoti Joshi, Direk Limmathurotsakul, and H. Rogier van Doorn. "Antimicrobial resistance surveillance in low-and middle-income countries: progress and challenges in eight South Asian and Southeast Asian countries." *Clinical Microbiology Reviews* 33, no. 3 (2020): e00048-19.

[22] Limmathurotsakul, D., Dunachie, S., Fukuda, K., Feasey, N. A., Okeke, I. N., Holmes, A. H., Moore, C. E., Dolecek, C., van Doorn, H. R., Shetty, N., Lopez, A. D., & Peacock, S. J. "Improving the estimation of the global burden of antimicrobial resistant infections." *The Lancet Infectious Diseases* 19, no. 11 (2019): e392-e398.

[23] Jonas, Olga B., Alec Irwin, Franck Cesar Jean Berthe, Francois G. Le Gall, and Patricio V. Marquez. "Drug-resistant infections: a threat to our economic future (Vol. 2): final report." *HNP/Agriculture Global Antimicrobial Resistance Initiative* (2017).

[24] Sandra Ponen, w.h.o., https://www.healthnavigator.org.nz/medicines/a/antibiotic-resistance/#Overview. 2017.

[25] Reygaert, Wanda C. "An overview of the antimicrobial resistance mechanisms of bacteria." *AIMS Microbiology* 4, no. 3 (2018): 482.

[26] Andersson, Dan I., and Diarmaid Hughes. "Selection and transmission of antibiotic-resistant bacteria." *Microbiology Spectrum* 5, no. 4 (2017): 5-4.

[27] World Health Organization, *WHO Publishes List of Bacteria for Which New Antibiotics are Urgently Needed.* 2017.

[28] Munkholm, L. and O. Rubin, The global governance of antimicrobial resistance: a cross-country study of alignment between the global action plan and national action plans. *Globalization and Health*, 2020. 16(1): p. 109.

[29] Zrnčić, S. N. J. E. Ž. A. N. A. "European Union's Action Plan on Antimicrobial Resistance and Implications for Trading Partners with Example of National Action Plan for Croatia." *Asian Fish Sci. S* 33 (2020): 75-82.

[30] Sader, Helio S., Paul R. Rhomberg, Andrew S. Fuhrmeister, Rodrigo E. Mendes, Robert K. Flamm, and Ronald N. Jones. "Antimicrobial resistance surveillance and new drug development." In *Open Forum Infectious Diseases*, vol. 6, no. Supplement_1, pp. S5-S13. US: Oxford University Press, 2019.

[31] Núñez-Núñez, M., Navarro, M. D., Palomo, V., Rajendran, N. B., del Toro, M. D., Voss, A., Sharland, M., Sifakis, F., Tacconelli, E., Rodríguez-Baño, J., Burkert, F., Carrara, E., von Cube, M., Drgona, L., Gilchrist, K., Goossens, H., Harbarth, S., Hequet, D., Jafri, H., ... Zingg, W. "The methodology of surveillance for antimicrobial resistance and healthcare-associated infections in Europe (SUSPIRE): a systematic review of publicly available information." *Clinical Microbiology and Infection* 24, no. 2 (2018): 105-109.

[32] Gandra, Sumanth, Gerardo Alvarez-Uria, Paul Turner, Jyoti Joshi, Direk Limmathurotsakul, and H. Rogier van Doorn. "Antimicrobial resistance surveillance in low-and middle-income countries: progress and challenges in eight South Asian and Southeast Asian countries." *Clinical Microbiology Reviews* 33, no. 3 (2020): e00048-19.

[33] World Health Organisation., *Global antimicrobial resistance and use surveillance system (GLASS) report: 2021.*

[34] World Health Organisation., *Global antimicrobial resistance surveillance system (GLASS) report: early implementation 2017-2018.* 2018.

[35] AMBIDEXTROUS, BEING. "Stewardship for the 21st century." *Thinking* (2019).

[36] McGowan Jr, J. E., and D. N. Gerding. "Does antibiotic restriction prevent resistance?." *New Horizons (Baltimore, Md.)* 4, no. 3 (1996): 370-376.

[37] Singh, S., Menon, V. P., Mohamed, Z. U., Kumar, V. A., Nampoothiri, V., Sudhir, S., Moni, M., Dipu, T. S., Dutt, A., Edathadathil, F., Keerthivasan, G., Kaye, K. S., & Patel, P. K. "Implementation and impact of an antimicrobial stewardship program at a tertiary care center in South India." In *Open Forum Infectious Diseases*, vol. 6, no. 4, p. ofy290. US: Oxford University Press, 2019.

[38] Schuts, E. C., Hulscher, M. E. J. L., Mouton, J. W., Verduin, C. M., Stuart, J. W. T. C., Overdiek, H. W. P. M., van der Linden, P. D., Natsch, S., Hertogh, C. M. P. M., Wolfs, T. F. W., Schouten, J. A., Kullberg, B. J., & Prins, J. M. "Current evidence on hospital antimicrobial stewardship objectives: a systematic review and meta-analysis." *The Lancet Infectious Diseases* 16, no. 7 (2016): 847-856.

[39] Cox, Janneke Arnoldine, Erika Vlieghe, Marc Mendelson, Heiman Wertheim, L. Ndegwa, María Virginia Villegas, I. Gould, and G. Levy Hara. "Antibiotic stewardship in low-and middle-income countries: the same but different?." *Clinical Microbiology and Infection* 23, no. 11 (2017): 812-818.

[40] ReAct Report, *The World Needs New Antibiotics – So Why Aren't They Developed.* 2021.

[41] Davies, Julian. "Where have all the antibiotics gone?." *Canadian Journal of Infectious Diseases and Medical Microbiology* 17, no. 5 (2006): 287-290.

[42] Kållberg, Cecilia, Christine Årdal, Hege Salvesen Blix, Eili Klein, Elena M. Martinez, Morten Lindbæk, Kevin Outterson, John-Arne Røttingen, and Ramanan Laxminarayan. "Introduction and geographic availability of new antibiotics approved between 1999 and 2014." *PloS One* 13, no. 10 (2018): e0205166.

[43] Bawazir, Ali Mohammed Abdullah, and Manjula Shantaram Palaksha. "An Implication Of Actinomycetes On Human Well-Being: A Review." *Int J Pharm Pharm Sci* (2019).

[44] World Health Organisation, *Report on lack of new antibiotics threatens global efforts to contain drug-resistant infections.* 2020.

[45] Sharma, Priyanka, and Debajit Thakur. "Antimicrobial biosynthetic potential and diversity of culturable soil actinobacteria from forest ecosystems of Northeast India." *Scientific Reports* 10, no. 1 (2020): 1-18.

[46] Thakur, D., A. Yadav, B. K. Gogoi, and T. C. Bora. "Isolation and screening of Streptomyces in soil of protected forest areas from the states of Assam and Tripura, India, for antimicrobial metabolites." *Journal de Mycologie Médicale* 17, no. 4 (2007): 242-249.

[47] Miao, Vivian, and Julian Davies. "Actinobacteria: the good, the bad, and the ugly." *Antonie Van Leeuwenhoek* 98, no. 2 (2010): 143-150.

[48] Nguyen, Hue Thi, Anaya Raj Pokhrel, Chung Thanh Nguyen, Van Thuy Thi Pham, Dipesh Dhakal, Haet Nim Lim, Hye Jin Jung, Tae-Su Kim, Tokutaro Yamaguchi, and Jae Kyung Sohng. "Streptomyces sp. VN1, a producer of diverse metabolites including non-natural furan-type anticancer compound." *Scientific Reports* 10, no. 1 (2020): 1-14.

[49] Nair, Soumya, and Jayanthi Abraham. "Natural products from actinobacteria for drug discovery." In *Advances in Pharmaceutical Biotechnology*, pp. 333-363. Springer, Singapore, 2020.

[50] Huan, Yuchen, Qing Kong, Haijin Mou, and Huaxi Yi. "Antimicrobial peptides: classification, design, application and research progress in multiple fields." *Frontiers in Microbiology* (2020): 2559.

[51] Wang, Guangshun. "Database-guided discovery of potent peptides to combat HIV-1 or superbugs." *Pharmaceuticals* 6, no. 6 (2013): 728-758.

[52] Divyashree, Mithoor, Madhu K. Mani, Dhanasekhar Reddy, Ranjith Kumavath, Preetam Ghosh, Vasco Azevedo, and Debmalya Barh. "Clinical applications of antimicrobial peptides (AMPs): where do we stand now?." *Protein and Peptide Letters* 27, no. 2 (2020): 120-134.

[53] León-Buitimea, Angel, Cesar R. Garza-Cárdenas, Javier A. Garza-Cervantes, Jordy A. Lerma-Escalera, and Jose R. Morones-Ramírez. "The demand for new

antibiotics: antimicrobial peptides, nanoparticles, and combinatorial therapies as future strategies in antibacterial agent design." *Frontiers in Microbiology* (2020): 1669.

[54] Zharkova, Maria S., Dmitriy S. Orlov, Olga Yu Golubeva, Oleg B. Chakchir, Igor E. Eliseev, Tatyana M. Grinchuk, and Olga V. Shamova. "Application of antimicrobial peptides of the innate immune system in combination with conventional antibiotics—a novel way to combat antibiotic resistance?." *Frontiers in Cellular and Infection Microbiology* 9 (2019): 128.

[55] Akbari, Reza, Mojdeh Hakemi-Vala, Fatemeh Pashaie, Parvaneh Bevalian, Ali Hashemi, and Kamran Pooshang Bagheri. "Highly synergistic effects of melittin with conventional antibiotics against multidrug-resistant isolates of acinetobacter baumannii and pseudomonas aeruginosa." *Microbial Drug Resistance* 25, no. 2 (2019): 193-202.

[56] Li, C., Zhu, C., Ren, B., Yin, X., Shim, S. H., Gao, Y., Zhu, J., Zhao, P., Liu, C., Yu, R., Xia, X., & Zhang, L. "Two optimized antimicrobial peptides with therapeutic potential for clinical antibiotic-resistant Staphylococcus aureus." *European Journal of Medicinal Chemistry* 183 (2019): 111686.

[57] Wang, Linlin, Chen Hu, and Longquan Shao. "The antimicrobial activity of nanoparticles: present situation and prospects for the future." *International Journal of Nanomedicine* 12 (2017): 1227.

[58] Santos, C. L., A. J. R. Albuquerque, F. C. Sampaio, and D. Keyson. "Nanomaterials with antimicrobial properties: applications in health sciences." *Microbial Pathogens and Strategies for Combating Them: Science, Technology and Education.* Volume 4, no. 2 (2013).

[59] Mazumdar, Rajkumari, and Debajit Thakur. "Therapeutic Applications of Nanotechnology in the Prevention of Infectious Diseases." In *Emerging Nanomaterials for Advanced Technologies*, pp. 323-343. Springer, Cham, 2022.

[60] Patra, J. K., Das, G., Fraceto, L. F., Campos, E. V. R., Rodriguez-Torres, M. del P., Acosta-Torres, L. S., Diaz-Torres, L. A., Grillo, R., Swamy, M. K., Sharma, S., Habtemariam, S., & Shin, H. S. "Nano based drug delivery systems: recent developments and future prospects." *Journal of Nanobiotechnology* 16, no. 1 (2018): 1-33.

[61] Ramalingam, Baskaran, Thanusu Parandhaman, and Sujoy K. Das. "Antibacterial effects of biosynthesized silver nanoparticles on surface ultrastructure and nanomechanical properties of gram-negative bacteria viz. Escherichia coli and Pseudomonas aeruginosa." *ACS Applied Materials & Interfaces* 8, no. 7 (2016): 4963-4976.

[62] Nas, F. S., M. Ali, and A. Muhammad. "Application of nanomaterials as antimicrobial agents: a review." *Archives of Nanomedicine* 1, no. 3 (2018): 59-64.

[63] Sobhani, Zahra, Soliman Mohammadi Samani, Hashem Montaseri, and Elham Khezri. "Nanoparticles of chitosan loaded ciprofloxacin: fabrication and antimicrobial activity." *Advanced Pharmaceutical Bulletin* 7, no. 3 (2017): 427.

[64] McMillan, JoEllyn, Elena Batrakova, and Howard E. Gendelman. "Cell delivery of therapeutic nanoparticles." *Progress in Molecular Biology and Translational Science* 104 (2011): 563-601.

Index

A

acid, vii, 2, 25, 27, 35, 37, 38, 39, 40, 41, 54, 55, 57, 58, 59, 60, 64, 66, 69, 71, 74, 75, 76, 77, 78, 81, 85, 86, 87, 88, 89, 90, 91, 92, 94, 95, 97, 102, 115, 116, 117, 118, 119, 183, 184, 209
actinobacteria, v, ix, 171, 172, 178, 179, 181, 182, 183, 185, 188, 189, 192, 193, 194, 195, 198, 209, 210, 216
advancements, ix, 84, 175, 198
adverse effects, 5, 8, 33, 53, 56
Africa, 7, 8, 9, 11, 12, 13, 14, 15, 20, 63, 82, 203, 207
age, 6, 20, 23, 208
agent-based model, vii, 124, 126, 168
agriculture, 175, 179, 180
AIDS, 2, 6, 28, 42, 47, 59, 106, 174
airports, viii, 124, 163, 164, 166
ammonium, 25, 27, 98, 99
antibiotic resistance, vii, ix, 105, 118, 175, 176, 177, 186, 187, 198, 199, 203, 204, 205, 206, 208, 212, 213, 217
antibiotics, v, vii, ix, 3, 4, 7, 10, 82, 83, 84, 85, 86, 87, 88, 89, 90, 91, 104, 105, 118, 172, 175, 176, 177, 178, 179, 180, 181, 182, 183, 184, 185, 186, 187, 188, 189, 190, 191, 192, 197, 198, 202, 203, 204, 205, 206, 207, 208, 209, 210, 211, 212, 213, 214, 215,216, 217
antibodies, v, vii, viii, 47, 96, 97, 98, 123, 124, 126, 127, 128, 129, 131, 132, 133, 137, 138, 141, 142, 143, 150, 152, 154, 155, 156, 157, 158, 159, 161, 162, 163, 165, 166, 168, 169
antigen, 53, 92, 95, 96, 97, 99, 101, 120
antimicrobial peptides, 198, 210, 216, 217
antimicrobial resistance, 104, 185, 198, 205, 206, 208, 213, 214, 215
antiviral agents, 42, 43, 176, 185
antiviral drugs, 42, 53, 112, 184
antiviral therapy, 42, 112, 114
Asia, 8, 11, 12, 13, 14, 15, 20, 203
asymptomatic, 10, 11, 13, 14, 15, 19
ATO, 25, 35, 36, 37, 38, 39, 40, 41, 54, 55, 56, 57, 58, 60, 61, 73, 74, 75, 76, 81, 85, 86, 87, 89, 91, 98
awareness, 175, 200, 205

B

bacteria, ix, 3, 6, 15, 82, 83, 104, 173, 175, 176, 178, 179, 180, 181, 182, 183, 185, 186, 189, 192, 197, 198, 202, 203, 204, 205, 208, 211, 212, 213, 215, 217
bacterial infection, 10, 17, 176, 198, 203, 212
bacterial pathogens, 176, 182, 198
bacterial strains, 84, 176, 203, 205, 208, 209, 211
bacterium, 20, 198, 203
barriers, 8, 93, 186
base, 22, 95, 96, 102, 103, 115, 116, 149, 201
bioactive metabolites, vii, ix, 172, 178, 180, 184
bioavailability, 4, 5, 8, 26, 32, 33, 34, 36, 41, 52, 53, 54, 57, 58, 60, 64, 74, 76, 80, 81, 82, 83, 84, 85, 87, 88, 89, 90, 105, 106, 109, 112, 113, 114, 117
biological activity, 120, 180, 189, 192
biomaterials, vii, 1, 2, 5, 6, 26, 94, 120

biomolecules, 26, 33, 34, 93, 94
biotechnology, 186, 188, 189, 194, 195
blood, 9, 18, 19, 22, 49, 56, 57, 77, 83, 87, 106, 117, 204, 205
blood-brain barrier, 22, 56, 57, 106
bloodstream, 63, 64, 75, 83, 198, 199, 205
bone, 20, 70, 98
brain, 17, 19, 53, 56, 57, 58, 59, 62, 64, 79, 82, 83, 87, 88, 105, 108, 112, 113, 116, 117

C

cancer, 4, 24, 28, 92, 105, 174, 180, 184, 199
candidates, 92, 183, 189
Carbopol, 36, 38, 39, 40
castor oil, 60, 74, 115
Center for Disease Control (CDC), 108, 114, 176
cell line, 96, 112, 118
cell membranes, 67, 93, 94, 212
central nervous system (CNS), 13, 19, 22, 52, 83, 106, 107, 112, 198
challenges, ix, 5, 21, 84, 93, 102, 107, 119, 197, 214, 215
chemical, 26, 81, 119, 178, 180, 189, 190, 209
chemotherapy, 7, 116, 186, 203, 211
children, 18, 20, 63, 174, 175
China, 84, 124, 207
chitosan, 77, 78, 83, 86, 117, 119, 217
cholesterol, 25, 40, 60, 79, 95, 99, 100, 113
choline, 25, 27, 79
circulation, 21, 52, 63, 64, 74
classes, 94, 130, 176, 177, 185
clinical trials, vii, 2, 22, 93, 101, 102, 103, 108
commercial, 33, 62, 63, 76, 79, 93, 98, 102, 103, 163, 164, 166, 192, 193
community, 3, 8, 18, 20, 174, 177, 186, 194
compliance, 8, 39, 52, 78, 83
composition, 22, 25, 34, 53, 82, 84, 119
compounds, ix, 25, 32, 172, 177, 178, 180, 182, 183, 185, 188, 189, 209, 214
contaminated food, 63, 172, 173, 198
convergence, viii, 123, 124, 126, 128, 129, 136, 138, 139, 140, 149, 154, 157, 159, 160, 161, 162, 163, 165, 166
cost, 8, 18, 24, 27, 29, 39, 84, 92, 176, 185, 203
cough, 12, 49, 51, 127, 138
COVID-19, viii, 4, 6, 7, 23, 24, 42, 84, 93, 94, 101, 106, 118, 124, 166, 167, 171, 174, 190
culture, 75, 182, 183, 184, 187
cytotoxicity, 24, 79, 81, 85, 86, 89, 95, 97, 99, 112, 114, 211

D

death, vii, 1, 2, 6, 11, 17, 19, 29, 66, 75, 83, 104, 129, 135, 142, 173, 174, 176, 198, 199, 203, 212
degradation, 24, 26, 70, 82, 94, 96, 102
developed countries, 2, 63, 175, 200
developing countries, 2, 8, 21, 64, 82, 104, 175
diarrhea, 18, 19, 43, 44, 45, 48, 49, 51
diffusion, 3, 27, 35, 41, 56, 60, 63, 85, 90
disability, 9, 14, 15, 20, 173
diseases, vii, viii, ix, 1, 2, 3, 4, 5, 6, 7, 8, 9, 10, 13, 15, 18, 20, 22, 23, 24, 28, 29, 32, 43, 50, 63, 82, 83, 84, 92, 93, 101, 102, 103, 106, 107, 108, 114, 125, 171, 172, 173, 174, 175, 176, 177, 181, 184, 185, 186, 187, 188, 190, 197, 198, 199, 203, 205, 211, 212, 214, 215
dispersion, 25, 29, 30, 57, 74, 87
distribution, 12, 42, 53, 56, 62, 88, 114, 117
diversity, 178, 189, 190, 216
dizziness, 19, 43, 44, 45, 46, 47, 49
DNA, 43, 44, 45, 47, 48, 51, 53, 67, 68, 72, 92, 93, 94, 95, 96, 99, 100, 102, 118, 119, 120, 121, 192
DNA polymerase, 43, 47, 48
DNA vaccines, 92, 93, 96, 118

dosage, 33, 39, 78, 179
dosing, 33, 52, 83
drug delivery, vii, 1, 2, 4, 5, 23, 24, 25, 26, 28, 33, 34, 35, 38, 54, 56, 57, 64, 73, 85, 103, 105, 108, 109, 110, 113, 115, 120, 211, 217
drug discovery, 103, 187, 216
drug release, 2, 4, 26, 36, 37, 38, 39, 52, 54, 56, 58, 73, 77, 85, 110, 112, 212
drug resistance, 2, 3, 32, 176, 185, 187, 195, 204, 205, 211, 212
drug targeting, vii, 1, 5, 22, 76, 83, 106
drugs, vii, 1, 2, 4, 5, 6, 7, 8, 13, 21, 22, 25, 26, 27, 28, 29, 32, 34, 40, 42, 52, 53, 59, 63, 64, 65, 67, 68, 69, 71, 72, 75, 77, 78, 79, 82, 83, 84, 85, 95, 102, 103, 104, 105, 108, 110, 112, 116, 177, 184, 188, 198, 203, 204, 208, 209, 210, 211

E

ecosystems, ix, 172, 174, 179, 195, 198, 216
edema, 10, 19, 43, 50, 51
education, 11, 18, 20, 217
egg, 25, 35, 55, 61
encapsulation, 6, 26, 64, 73, 103
encoding, 67, 94, 95, 98, 99, 100, 101, 102, 121
endophytes, 178, 179, 180, 183, 184, 185, 187, 188
endophytic actinobacteria (EA), vii, ix, 112, 172, 178, 181, 183, 185, 186, 188, 190, 192, 193
energy, 27, 67, 72
environment, ix, 3, 13, 16, 20, 94, 172, 173, 178, 179, 185, 197, 198, 206, 212
enzyme, 30, 31, 42, 67, 72, 81, 184, 185
epidemic, 126, 167, 174
Europe, 10, 11, 188, 215
evaporation, 27, 35, 40, 41, 55, 56, 59, 61, 77, 78, 80, 81, 86, 89, 91
evidence, 34, 179, 200, 201, 215
evolution, ix, 7, 64, 172, 174
exposure, 6, 14, 77, 188, 204

F

Food and Drug Administration (FDA), vii, 2, 4, 22, 23, 24, 30, 31, 43, 44, 45, 46, 47, 48, 49, 50, 51, 65, 66, 67, 68, 69, 70, 71, 72, 94, 103
FDA approval, 22, 30, 31, 43, 44, 45, 46, 47, 48, 49, 50, 51, 65, 66, 67, 68, 69, 70, 71, 72
fever, viii, 7, 10, 11, 12, 49, 82, 123, 124, 126, 132, 156, 157, 159, 161, 162, 164, 165, 213
fluid, 27, 73, 85
food, 3, 11, 19, 63, 83, 172, 173, 185, 188, 198, 206
fungal infection, 16, 23, 29, 30, 32, 33, 34, 38, 108, 109, 176
fungi, 15, 29, 173, 179, 180, 181, 182, 183, 187, 188, 189, 192

G

gel, 36, 40, 41, 110, 111
gene therapy, 4, 92, 119
genes, 50, 70, 94, 95, 106, 176, 178, 189, 190
genome, 72, 92, 93, 179
genus, 13, 178, 181, 189
glycerol, 25, 55, 60, 85, 95, 97
glycol, 36, 62, 89, 95, 98, 105
growth, 18, 63, 72, 80, 85, 126, 175, 179, 187, 192, 193, 194, 204, 212

H

habitats, 180, 185, 209
half-life, 52, 77, 82, 92
HBV (hepatitis B virus), 42, 43, 48, 50, 51, 53, 56, 96, 112
headache, 43, 44, 45, 48, 49, 50, 51
health, viii, ix, 2, 3, 6, 8, 11, 17, 18, 20, 28, 29, 42, 83, 104, 112, 114, 171, 172, 173, 174, 176, 179, 180, 185, 187, 188, 197, 198, 199, 200, 201, 202, 203, 204, 206, 207, 208, 213, 217
health care, 3, 17, 29, 201, 202, 206, 213

Helicobacter pylori, 95, 99, 102, 205
hepatitis, 23, 42, 96, 112, 120, 174
history, 7, 21, 84, 173, 185, 203, 209, 213
HIV, 2, 5, 6, 28, 42, 44, 45, 46, 47, 48, 51, 52, 53, 57, 59, 93, 99, 100, 105, 106, 112, 113, 120, 184, 216
HIV-1, 44, 45, 46, 47, 93, 106, 112, 184, 216
host, ix, 3, 4, 5, 13, 42, 45, 49, 66, 79, 92, 93, 94, 102, 111, 126, 127, 172, 173, 178, 179, 180, 193, 210
human, viii, ix, 3, 6, 7, 17, 18, 28, 34, 42, 63, 70, 92, 99, 101, 103, 108, 112, 127, 159, 162, 171, 172, 173, 174, 175, 180, 181, 182, 184, 188, 198, 203, 204
human health, viii, 42, 171, 180, 188, 204
hygiene, 7, 19, 200, 201, 213
hypersensitivity, 43, 44, 45

I

identification, 166, 186, 189, 190
immune cells, vii, 50, 99, 124, 126, 127, 128, 129, 131, 132, 133, 136, 138, 156, 158, 159, 161, 165
immune response, viii, 3, 16, 80, 92, 95, 96, 97, 98, 100, 102, 120, 123, 126, 127, 141, 142, 161, 162, 165
immune system, 42, 52, 126, 158, 159, 161, 166, 210, 217
immunity, viii, 96, 98, 100, 121, 123, 132, 139, 141, 142, 156, 157, 159, 161, 162, 163, 165, 166, 167, 173
immunization, ix, 6, 7, 47, 120, 197
immunocompromised, 3, 28, 29
immunodeficiency, 51, 174, 184
immunogenicity, 92, 94, 102
improvements, 7, 103, 212
in vitro, 33, 41, 52, 55, 61, 73, 76, 78, 80, 82, 95, 96, 100, 109, 110, 112, 115, 116, 117, 118, 120, 211
in vivo, 36, 38, 42, 53, 73, 76, 80, 82, 94, 95, 105, 109, 110, 111, 115, 117, 118, 211
incidence, 29, 87, 102, 173, 184, 200
income, 2, 10, 63, 200, 201, 214, 215, 216
India, 171, 184, 188, 191, 192, 193, 194, 195, 197, 207, 213, 215, 216
individuals, viii, 15, 28, 123, 124, 150, 153, 160, 162, 163, 164, 165, 166, 174
induction, 96, 97, 193
industry, 173, 175, 177, 179, 180, 182, 206
influenza, 23, 93, 111, 175, 181, 184
ingestion, 11, 12, 18, 19
inhibition, 43, 68, 69, 70, 71, 72, 85, 100, 106, 212
inhibitor, 47, 51, 53, 112, 184, 186
insomnia, 44, 45, 48, 49
integration, 45, 93, 96
investment, 8, 21, 205, 208
Iran, 111, 115, 189
isolation, viii, ix, 123, 124, 163, 166, 172, 179, 182, 186, 188, 189, 190, 209, 213, 216
isoniazid, 85, 87, 117
issues, 21, 52, 104, 179

J

Japan, 123, 148, 149, 168

K

kill, 28, 64, 198, 203, 212

L

lactic acid, 43, 75, 115
lactose, 25, 78, 97
larvae, 10, 15, 189
lead, 18, 20, 27, 64, 179, 184
lecithin, 25, 27, 36, 40, 41, 54, 56, 58, 61, 62, 73, 74, 76, 77, 79, 80, 87, 90
leishmaniasis, 23, 63, 68, 79, 80, 84, 100, 102, 103, 116, 121
lesions, 9, 16, 19, 67, 192
light, 6, 28, 92
lipids, 24, 25, 26, 27, 28, 38, 107
liposomes, 4, 24, 95, 103, 107, 212
liver, 11, 12, 26, 43, 64, 70, 87, 88, 90, 105, 174

lymph, 64, 75, 113, 115

M

macrophages, 21, 46, 50, 52, 59, 79, 80, 83, 85, 90, 105, 107, 113, 117
majority, 163, 175, 178, 198, 208
malaria, 2, 28, 63, 77, 82, 84, 103, 173, 175, 213
management, ix, 13, 64, 102, 115, 117, 168, 193, 198, 200, 201, 202, 207
manufacturing, 92, 93, 95
masks, viii, 124, 127, 132, 147, 165
materials, 21, 28, 211, 217
matrix, vii, 1, 3, 24, 25, 26, 33, 49, 74
matter, 2, 21, 28, 94
meat, 175, 184, 186
media, 3, 92, 173, 174
medical, 3, 8, 21, 104, 126, 172, 175, 177, 179, 190, 199, 201, 203
medicine, 4, 6, 21, 84, 114, 166, 172, 179, 180, 184, 189, 198, 213, 214
Mediterranean, 11, 13, 14, 188
membranes, 14, 67, 93, 94, 198, 212
meta-analysis, 190, 214, 215
metabolism, 53, 57, 63, 64, 66, 68, 72, 87, 178, 185
metabolites, vii, ix, 172, 178, 179, 180, 182, 183, 184, 185, 187, 188, 189, 192, 195, 209, 216
mice, 53, 73, 78, 80, 87, 97, 98, 100, 102, 109, 114, 115, 116, 121
microbes, 177, 178, 179, 184, 190, 192, 198, 204, 210
microemulsion, 27, 54, 74, 79, 111
microorganisms, ix, 3, 4, 5, 6, 15, 22, 92, 102, 172, 173, 176, 177, 178, 179, 180, 197, 198
models, 114, 124, 125, 126
molecular weight, 78, 86, 102
molecules, vii, ix, 1, 32, 78, 93, 94, 95, 96, 172, 177, 184, 190
morbidity, 2, 9, 11, 18, 28, 102, 175, 176, 199, 200, 212
mortality, 2, 28, 42, 63, 82, 102, 175, 176, 199, 200, 208, 212
mRNA, 4, 6, 23, 24, 49, 92, 93, 94, 95, 96, 98, 101, 102, 118, 119, 120, 121
myalgia, 43, 49, 50

N

nanomaterials, vii, 2, 21, 104, 212, 217
nanomedicine, 21, 22, 103, 217
nanoparticles (NPs), vii, 1, 2, 4, 5, 6, 21, 22, 23, 24, 25, 26, 27, 28, 32, 33, 34, 35, 38, 39, 40, 41, 42, 52, 53, 54, 55, 56, 57, 58, 59, 60, 61, 62, 63, 64, 73, 74, 75, 78, 79, 80, 81, 82, 83, 84, 85, 86, 87, 93, 94, 95, 96, 97, 98, 99, 100, 102, 103, 104, 105, 106, 107, 108, 109, 110, 111, 112, 113, 114, 115, 116, 117, 118, 119, 120, 121, 198, 211, 212, 217
nanotechnology, vii, 1, 4, 5, 6, 8, 21, 24, 63, 83, 104
national borders, viii, 124, 163, 164, 166
nausea, 43, 44, 45, 47, 48, 49, 50
neglected tropical diseases, 2, 5, 9, 24, 107
nervous system, 13, 19, 22, 107, 198
nucleic acid, 69, 71, 92, 93, 94, 95, 102, 119, 120

O

oil, 24, 27, 59, 60, 74, 77, 84, 90, 115, 179
optimization, 111, 112, 113, 116, 117, 189
organ, 5, 9, 21, 28, 42, 52, 59, 83, 88, 94, 103, 198, 199, 200, 202
organism, 172, 178, 179, 212
otitis media, 3, 173, 174

P

Pacific, 14, 15, 20, 207
pain, 10, 11, 18, 19, 43, 45, 46, 47, 48, 49, 50, 51
pandemic, viii, 6, 42, 84, 93, 106, 112, 123, 124, 125, 128, 133, 139, 140, 141, 143, 148, 149, 150, 152, 154, 155, 156, 157,

158, 159, 160, 161, 162, 163, 165, 166, 171, 174, 176
pandemic convergence, viii, 123, 128, 140, 154, 157, 159, 160, 161, 162, 163, 165, 166
parasite, 10, 11, 12, 13, 63, 64, 66, 68, 69, 70, 72, 75, 77, 80, 100, 114
pathogenesis, vii, 1, 4, 213
pathogenic bacteria, ix, 82, 175, 197, 198, 204, 211
pathogenic microorganisms, ix, 173, 197, 198
pathogens, ix, 2, 3, 4, 5, 7, 92, 96, 108, 109, 172, 174, 175, 176, 177, 179, 180, 181, 182, 184, 185, 193, 195, 199, 203, 207, 209, 212, 217
pathways, 50, 67, 181, 186, 190
PCR tests, viii, 123, 163, 164
penicillin, 7, 20, 179, 181, 185, 190, 191, 202, 205, 208
peptides, vii, 1, 25, 95, 120, 180, 181, 182, 184, 187, 198, 210, 211, 216, 217
permeability, 35, 39, 53, 61, 76, 77, 82, 86, 115
permeation, 38, 40, 53, 55, 89, 111, 115
pharmaceutical, 8, 21, 32, 33, 103, 177, 180, 182, 185, 190, 208, 209, 210, 217
pharmacokinetics, 112, 115, 117
phosphatidylcholine, 29, 35, 38, 55, 61, 75, 88, 91
physicochemical properties, 22, 25, 32, 34, 53, 82, 84, 94, 107, 110, 118, 211
plants, 12, 53, 178, 179, 180, 181, 182, 185, 187, 190, 193, 211
plasmid DNA, 93, 96, 118, 119
platform, 92, 93, 95, 96, 103
PM, 116, 117, 120
pneumonia, 3, 21, 82, 174, 186, 198, 200, 204
polydispersity, 25, 27, 28
polymer, 22, 24, 86, 103, 212
polymerase, 43, 47, 48, 49, 69, 70, 71
polyvinyl alcohol, 25, 35, 41, 59, 60, 61, 74, 75, 76, 77, 78, 85, 86, 89
population, 15, 28, 129, 133, 143, 157, 176, 204, 206, 207
poverty, ix, 3, 8, 18, 172, 185
preparation, vii, 2, 6, 26, 27, 34, 35, 36, 37, 38, 39, 40, 41, 53, 54, 55, 56, 57, 58, 59, 60, 61, 62, 73, 74, 75, 76, 77, 78, 79, 80, 81, 82, 83, 84, 85, 86, 87, 88, 89, 90, 91, 97, 98, 99, 100, 115, 118
prevention, vii, 4, 7, 19, 23, 29, 34, 41, 53, 57, 102, 113, 147, 152, 176, 184, 200, 202, 203, 205, 206, 208, 213, 214
probability, 124, 144, 146, 150, 154, 160, 163, 164, 165
pro-inflammatory, 30, 96, 99
proliferation, 67, 96, 98
prophylaxis, v, vii, 1, 2, 9, 10, 11, 12, 13, 14, 15, 16, 17, 18, 19, 20, 92
propylene, 36, 89, 105
protection, 10, 15, 25, 97
protein synthesis, 68, 69, 71
proteins, vii, 1, 22, 34, 45, 46, 50, 67, 95, 96, 100, 101, 107, 120
pruritus, 10, 17, 45, 50
Pseudomonas aeruginosa, 89, 180, 202, 205, 211, 212, 214, 217
public health, viii, ix, 11, 29, 83, 171, 173, 174, 176, 197, 198, 202, 206, 212
pumps, 34, 52, 106

R

rash, 44, 45, 46, 47, 48, 50
reactions, 30, 31, 46, 47, 48, 50
receptors, 21, 46, 47, 65, 66, 82, 83
recovery, vii, 79, 120, 123, 124, 125, 126, 132, 136, 138, 139, 141, 142, 150, 154, 155, 157, 160, 161, 163, 166, 173
relaxation, 132, 150, 151, 152
replication, viii, 42, 46, 50, 53, 68, 72, 123, 126, 127, 128, 129, 131, 132, 133, 134, 135, 136, 137, 138, 139, 140, 141, 142, 143, 144, 145, 146, 147, 150, 151, 152, 153, 154, 155, 156, 157, 158, 159, 161, 162, 163, 165, 173

resistance, vii, ix, 2, 3, 5, 8, 25, 32, 42, 64, 69, 104, 105, 106, 107, 109, 112, 118, 172, 175, 176, 177, 180, 185, 186, 187, 189, 198, 203, 204, 205, 206, 207, 208, 212, 213, 214, 215, 217
resources, 29, 195, 201, 208
response, viii, 16, 42, 54, 66, 80, 92, 95, 96, 97, 100, 120, 123, 126, 127, 141, 142, 161, 162, 165, 173, 208
restrictions, 124, 132, 150, 151, 152, 163
risk, 15, 18, 82, 95, 96, 102, 173, 176, 186, 188, 200, 212
RNA, 49, 68, 92, 93, 94, 95, 118, 121, 192
roots, 178, 180, 189
routes, 4, 32, 36, 37, 83, 95, 96

S

safety, 33, 39, 41, 79, 89, 92, 94, 117
Salmonella, 4, 82, 83, 99, 184, 186, 198
SARS-CoV-2, 6, 42, 84, 93, 94, 118, 124, 148, 167
scabies, 76, 82, 84
schistosomiasis, 18, 63, 84, 115
science, 6, 114, 168, 217
sepsis, 10, 200, 214
serum, 22, 57, 98
shear, 27, 35, 40, 59, 75, 79, 90, 100
showing, 141, 157, 158, 159, 161, 204
side effects, 30, 31, 32, 39, 42, 64, 80, 82, 84, 92, 102, 118
silver, 5, 212, 217
siRNA, 95, 102, 119
skin, 9, 10, 14, 17, 20, 28, 33, 35, 36, 38, 39, 40, 41, 46, 48, 50, 55, 82, 173, 198
sodium, 23, 25, 29, 30, 35, 38, 40, 54, 55, 60, 61, 69, 72, 74, 75, 77, 78, 79, 85, 88, 89, 90, 97, 100
solid lipid nanoparticles (SLNs), vii, 1, 2, 5, 6, 22, 24, 25, 26, 27, 28, 32, 33, 34, 35, 38, 39, 40, 41, 42, 52, 53, 54, 55, 56, 57, 58, 59, 60, 61, 62, 63, 64, 73, 74, 75, 78, 79, 80, 81, 82, 83, 84, 85, 86, 87, 95, 96, 97, 99, 100, 102, 103, 104, 106, 108, 109, 110, 111, 112, 113, 114, 115, 116, 117, 118, 119, 120, 121
solidification, 35, 54, 168
solubility, 4, 21, 26, 27, 32, 64, 76, 78, 82, 83, 90, 103
solution, 8, 25, 29, 30, 53, 61, 79, 87, 177
South America, 7, 8, 11, 12, 15, 20
Southeast Asia, 13, 14, 20, 214, 215
species, 5, 7, 10, 18, 28, 29, 63, 102, 111, 174, 179, 181, 183, 186, 194, 198
spleen, 26, 88, 90
stability, 4, 24, 25, 26, 27, 36, 40, 54, 55, 58, 59, 73, 76, 78, 81, 92, 95, 96, 105, 110, 115, 212
states, vii, 2, 32, 52, 126, 128, 130, 131, 132, 161, 174, 176, 206, 216
stewardship, v, vii, 197, 207, 208, 215, 216
storage, 25, 27, 92, 95
structure, 26, 28, 109, 125, 169
sub-Saharan Africa, 20, 63, 82
sulfate, 29, 60, 75, 79, 100, 109, 117
sun, 118, 187, 190
surfactant, 22, 25, 27, 28, 107, 117
surveillance, 104, 109, 199, 200, 201, 205, 206, 213, 214, 215
survival, 3, 67, 178
sustained drug release, 2, 4, 38, 39, 77
symptoms, ix, 12, 17, 18, 19, 46, 49, 50, 197
synthesis, 31, 43, 44, 47, 49, 68, 69, 71, 114, 178, 180, 192, 209

T

T cell, 50, 96, 98, 101, 120
target, 4, 21, 22, 40, 42, 53, 64, 94, 96, 103, 184, 186, 188, 208, 211
targeted drug delivery, 2, 5, 25, 212
techniques, ix, 4, 27, 28, 93, 197
technologies, 4, 8, 21, 84, 92, 100, 102, 103, 168, 173, 177, 213, 217
temperature, viii, 22, 25, 27, 35, 54, 76, 92, 123, 124, 126, 127, 132, 161, 163, 164, 166, 167
therapeutic agents, 83, 177, 180

therapeutic approaches, 212
therapeutic effect, 4, 21, 38, 211
therapeutic use, 177, 178, 179
therapeutics, 8, 103, 108, 184, 188, 211
therapy, vii, 2, 4, 7, 14, 24, 29, 32, 39, 42, 53, 63, 64, 83, 84, 89, 92, 105, 109, 112, 113, 114, 117, 119, 120, 213
tissue, 15, 16, 33, 117, 173, 178, 179, 198
toxicity, 5, 21, 22, 25, 26, 29, 32, 33, 41, 52, 54, 64, 73, 75, 78, 79, 82, 86, 87, 90, 94, 95, 102, 103, 115, 119, 212
transcription, 44, 68, 93, 182
transfection, 93, 94, 95, 100, 118, 119, 120
transformation, 26, 96, 174
transmission, 3, 14, 28, 53, 106, 111, 167, 172, 202, 212, 215
transport, 49, 53, 57, 65, 92, 93, 94, 114, 163, 166
treatment, v, vii, ix, 1, 3, 4, 8, 9, 10, 11, 17, 20, 21, 22, 24, 29, 30, 32, 33, 34, 37, 38, 39, 42, 43, 47, 52, 54, 59, 64, 76, 80, 82, 83, 87, 88, 102, 103, 109, 110, 115, 171, 172, 174, 176, 177, 184, 197, 199, 203, 204, 205, 208, 211, 212, 213
tuberculosis (TB), 2, 21, 28, 82, 83, 84, 85, 87, 88, 103, 116, 117, 173, 198, 203, 212, 213
two-dimensional space, 127, 129, 131, 132

U

uniform, 127, 129, 209
United States, 32, 174, 176
urinary tract infection, 195, 200, 205

V

vaccines, vii, 1, 2, 4, 6, 7, 10, 17, 23, 24, 42, 84, 92, 93, 94, 95, 96, 97, 98, 99, 100, 101, 102, 103, 106, 118, 119, 120, 121, 184, 188, 213
valuation, 73, 105, 111, 115, 117
vancomycin, 91, 205, 210
variables, 6, 110, 114, 125, 129, 130, 131, 132, 136
vector, 9, 13, 94, 114, 172
ventilation, viii, 124, 164
viral diseases, 10, 43, 93
viral infection, 42, 52, 96
viral particle, 49, 124, 127, 138, 147, 164, 165
viral vectors, 94, 95, 102, 119
virus, viii, 4, 7, 10, 23, 42, 43, 49, 51, 93, 94, 96, 98, 101, 102, 111, 112, 123, 124, 126, 127, 128, 129, 130, 131, 132, 133, 134, 135, 136, 137, 138, 139, 140, 141, 142, 143, 144, 145, 146, 147, 149, 150, 151, 152, 153, 154, 155, 156, 157, 158, 159, 160, 161, 162, 163, 164, 165, 166, 173, 174, 181, 184
virus replication, viii, 123, 128, 129, 131, 132, 133, 134, 135, 136, 137, 138, 139, 140, 141, 142, 143, 144, 145, 146, 147, 150, 151, 152, 153, 154, 155, 156, 157, 158, 159, 161, 162, 163, 165
vomiting, 43, 45, 48, 49, 50, 51

W

water, 8, 10, 11, 12, 18, 19, 25, 26, 33, 54, 74, 103, 113, 173, 179, 198
workers, 175, 201, 211
World Health Organization (WHO), vii, viii, 2, 3, 7, 63, 65, 82, 83, 84, 104, 106, 107, 116, 171, 174, 198, 199, 200, 201, 202, 204, 205, 206, 208, 213, 214, 215, 216
worldwide, vii, 1, 2, 9, 11, 12, 14, 15, 17, 18, 20, 28, 29, 63, 84, 124, 173, 174, 175, 177, 203, 213
worms, 17, 18, 63, 64, 173

Y

yeast, 23, 33, 34, 109, 179, 182, 211